Handbook of Fetal Medicine

Handbook of
Fetal Medicine

Sailesh Kumar
MBBS, M.Med(O&G), FRCS, FRCOG,
FRANZCOG, DPhil(Oxon), CMFM
Consultant and Senior Lecturer
Centre for Fetal & Maternal Medicine
Queen Charlotte's & Chelsea Hospital
Imperial College London

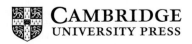
CAMBRIDGE
UNIVERSITY PRESS

CAMBRIDGE UNIVERSITY PRESS
Cambridge, New York, Melbourne, Madrid, Cape Town, Singapore,
São Paulo, Delhi, Dubai, Tokyo

Cambridge University Press
The Edinburgh Building, Cambridge CB2 8RU, UK

Published in the United States of America by
Cambridge University Press, New York

www.cambridge.org
Information on this title: www.cambridge.org/9780521675369

First published 2010

Printed in the United Kingdom at the University Press, Cambridge

A catalog record for this publication is available from the British Library

Library of Congress Cataloging-in-Publication data
Handbook of fetal medicine / edited by Sailesh Kumar.
    p. ; cm.
  Includes index.
  ISBN 978-0-521-67536-9 (pbk.)
  1. Perinatology–Handbooks, manuals, etc.   2. Fetus–Diseases–
Handbooks, manuals, etc. I. Kumar, Sailesh, 1966– II. Title.
  [DNLM: 1. Fetal Diseases–diagnosis.   2. Fetal Diseases–therapy.
3. Fetal Monitoring–methods.   4. Fetal Therapies–methods.
5. Fetus–physiology.   6. Prenatal Diagnosis–methods. WQ 211 H236 2010]
  RG600.H36 2010
  618.3'2–dc22

                     2010001105

ISBN 978-0-521-67536-9 Paperback

Dedicated to
Catherine, Radhika, Meera, Rahul, and Vikram

CONTENTS

Color plates will be found between pages 110 and 111.

PREFACE

Fetal medicine is now a well established subspecialty and is a vital part of any perinatal service. This field is huge and encompasses a wide range of conditions covering diverse areas ranging from genetics to perinatal pathology. Advances, particularly in the fields of non-invasive prenatal diagnosis and imaging, make this a constantly evolving specialty and an occasionally challenging one for the generalist obstetrician. Fetal medicine is very much a multidisciplinary specialty and it is imperative that anyone working in this area is sensitive to the fact that long-term outcome is not always predictable on antenatal imaging or testing and I hope that this is evident throughout the text.

A working knowledge of fetal medicine is essential for any obstetrician or obstetric physician and this book aims to provide a practical guide for clinicians of any grade who care for pregnant women with a fetal problem. It is by no means comprehensive, but hopefully covers many of the common important conditions encountered in clinical practice. The principles of management are discussed in broad detail in every chapter. Although the opinions contained within this book are a distillation of current published evidence and established practice, there is inevitably some personal preference and opinion that has influenced certain recommendations. I am grateful to all my colleagues for their support, but most importantly for their critical comments and advice.

I very much hope this handbook is useful to practicing clinicians who are involved in perinatal care and that it provides them with practical and sensible management options.

Sailesh Kumar
Queen Charlotte's & Chelsea Hospital
Imperial College London

GENETICS

Chromosome abnormalities and selected genetic syndromes

Modes of inheritance

Autosomal dominant (AD) inheritance

- These disorders are encoded on autosomes and will manifest when a single copy of the mutant allele is present (i.e. in heterozygotes). The disease/mutant allele is dominant to the wild-type allele.
- Males and females are equally affected and may both transmit the disease with a 50% risk of transmission to any offspring.
- Penetrance is the variability of clinical manifestation of an autosomal disorder. Many conditions (Huntington disease) show delayed or age-dependent penetrance in which the disease only becomes apparent after a period of time. Non-penetrance or incomplete penetrance occurs when an individual known to be heterozygous for the allele does not manifest the disease.
- The expressivity of the gene is the degree to which the particular disease manifests in affected individuals. In neurofibromatosis a mildly affected parent may have a child who is severely affected.
- New mutation rates vary significantly between AD conditions – 50% of cases of neurofibromatosis I are new mutations.
- A few AD dominant conditions (Huntington disease, myotonic dystrophy) demonstrate anticipation where there is worsening of the disease severity with each generation. This characteristically occurs in triplet repeat disorders when expansion of the triplet repeats occurs in either the maternal or paternal germline.
- In some cases of new dominant mutations there is a significant risk that a second child may be affected, despite both parents being normal. This is usually due to germline or gonadal mosaicism and can carry a high recurrence risk for some conditions (osteogenesis imperfecta type II).

Autosomal recessive (AR) inheritance

- Also encoded on the autosomes but only manifests in homozygotes or compound heterozygotes. Both parents are obligate carriers and will not usually have any manifestations of the disease. AR conditions are much more common in consanguineous families.
- Both males and females can be affected. The risk of having an affected child if both parents are carriers is 25%.
- Affected siblings generally show a similar clinical course, which is more consistent than for many AD conditions.

X-linked dominant (XLD) inheritance

- This is an uncommon form of inheritance and is caused by a dominant disease allele on the X chromosome. XLD disorders manifest very severely in males with spontaneous fetal loss or neonatal death commonly occurring.

- Female heterozygotes are less severely affected. The distribution of features in a female is a reflection of the X-inactivation pattern seen in specific tissues.
- Asymmetric involvement of the body is an important feature (e.g. in X-linked chondrodyplasia punctata, asymmetric limb shortening occurs).
- X inactivation in the embryo is a random process with 50% of cells containing the inactive maternal X chromosome and 50% containing the inactive paternal X chromosome.
- Significant deviation away from the normal 50:50 ratio is occasionally seen (skewed X inactivation).
- X-linked semi-dominant disorders manifest severely in males who are hemizygotes and mildly or subclinically in females who have two X chromosomes (normal and mutated copy).
- When an affected male reproduces, all female offspring will inherit the mutation but the male offspring will be unaffected. The family tree shows no male-to-male transmission.
- Females with severe features of an XLD disorder or an X-linked semi-dominant disorder may be affected because of highly unfavorable skewed X-inactivation, Turner syndrome (hemizygote) or X-autosome translocation.
- Males with features of a severe XLD disorder may have Klinefelter syndrome. Karyotyping is indicated in all cases.

X-linked recessive (XLR) inheritance

- XLR disorders manifests in males who are hemizygotes. Females are carriers because they carry two copies of the X chromosome (normal and mutant copy). Unfavorable skewing of X inactivation in key tissues is the main factor that determines whether or not a heterozygote expresses the disease.
- Some XLR conditions are never seen in females, whilst others have only infrequent symptoms (Duchenne and Becker muscular dystrophy). In other conditions (fragile X syndrome) carrier females are frequently symptomatic but never as severely affected as males.
- Duchenne and Becker muscular dystrophy have a significant risk of germline mosaicim.
- An affected male will father carrier daughters, but none of his sons will be affected. The family tree will show no male-to-male transmission.

Mitochondrial inheritance

- Mitochondrial DNA in humans is a double-stranded DNA encoding 13 proteins, 2 ribosomal RNAs and 22 transfer RNAs. Most of the mitochondrial genome is coding sequence.
- Tissues most often affected in mitochondrial disease are energy demanding organs (central nervous system, muscle, liver, and kidney). Preferential accumulation of mutant DNA in affected tissues explains the progressive nature of mitochondrial disorders.

1

- Mitochondrial DNA is maternal inherited except in very rare circumstances. Paternal mitochondria constitute only 0.1% of total mitochondria at fertilization and is rapidly eliminated. Males do not transmit mitochondrial disorders with very rare exceptions.
- A mitochondrial inherited condition can affect either sex. Human mitochondrial DNA has a much higher mutation rate (>10–$20\times$) than nuclear DNA.
- When a mutation arises in a cellular mitochondrial DNA, it creates the existence of both mutant and normal DNA. This is defined as heteroplasmy. In homoplasmy only one type of mitochondrial DNA is present (pure mutant or normal).
- If a mother is heteroplasmic for a particular mutation, the proportion of mutant DNA in her children may vary widely.
- The difference in mitochondrial function between normal and defective cells can be very small. This is called threshold expression.
- The available evidence suggests that there is little or no tissue variation in the mutant DNA in affected individuals. A prenatal sample from chorionic villous sampling (CVS)/amniocentesis therefore, can predict the mutant load in most tissues after birth, although trying to predict the phenotype from this is very difficult.

Multifactorial inheritance
- Many conditions depend on interaction between genetic factors and the environment to manifest. Diseases inherited this way are called complex diseases (diabetes mellitus, schizophrenia, ischemic heart disease) and are transmitted due to multifactorial inheritance.
- The mapping and identification of responsible genes is difficult because the candidate genes occur with similar frequency in affected and normal individuals.

Chromosomal abnormalities

Down syndrome (Trisomy 21)
- 95% of cases are the result of meiotic non-disjunction. 2% result from Robertsonian translocation (especially 14;21) of which 50% are familial. 2% of cases are due to mosaicism and 1% of cases occur from chromosome rearrangements. Trisomy for the 21q22 region results in many of the clinical features.
- The incidence increases with maternal age and there is a significant risk of fetal loss.
- 40%–50% of cases have cardiac abnormalities. Ventricular septal defect is the most common effect followed by patent ductus arteriosus. Atrioventricular septal defect (AVSD) is much more common in Down syndrome than in the general population.
- The risk of recurrence is influenced by maternal age and parental germline mosaicism. Overall, the risk of recurrence is approximately 1% for the common variant of Down syndrome.
- After two affected children, a recurrence risk of 10% may be more appropriate. If a previous child had a *de novo* Robertsonian

GENETICS

translocation, the risk of recurrence is low (<2% if parental chromosomes are normal).
- If the father carries a Robertsonian translocation involving chromosome 21, the recurrence risk is <1%. If the mother carries the translocation, the risk is 10%–15%.
- There are many different screening methods (combined test, integrated test, quadruple test, etc.) in low-risk pregnancies. Prenatal diagnosis is possible from any fetal sample (usually CVS or amniocentesis).

Edward syndrome (Trisomy 18)
- 94% of infants with Edward syndrome have trisomy 18. The remainder have trisomy 18 mosaicism or partial 18q trisomy. The majority of cases are due to meiotic non-disjunction. The risk increases with maternal age.
- Multiple fetal abnormalities are usually evident on antenatal ultrasound. There is an extremely high rate of fetal loss and the majority of live born infants die during the neonatal period.
- Prenatal diagnosis is possible from chorionic villi, amniocytes, or fetal blood.

Patau syndrome (Trisomy 13)
- 90% of cases are due to non-disjunction during meiosis, 5%–10% are caused by an unbalanced Robertsonian translocation (13;14) and a very small proportion is due to mosaicism. The risk increases with maternal age but the overall risk is still very low.
- The average survival is 7–10 days with the majority of pregnancies ending with fetal demise.
- Multiple fetal abnormalities are present on antenatal ultrasound and should prompt karyotyping.
- The overall recurrence risk is low (0.5%).
- Prenatal diagnosis is possible from any fetal sample.

22q11 deletion syndrome
- Also known as DiGeorge syndrome or velocardiofacial syndrome.
- 96% of cases have a defined microdeletion (1.5–3 Mb) of 22q11 which includes 24–30 genes.
- Cardiac defects, thymic hypoplasia, distinctive facial appearance, parathyroid insufficiency, and pharyngeal problems are part of the phenotypic spectrum.
- The phenotype arises from the failure of development of the third and fourth branchial arches. Haploinsufficiency of the *TBX1* gene is the major contributor to the phenotype.
- The diagnosis should be considered in any fetus with a cardiac abnormality particularly involving the outflow tracts. 75% of cases have congenital heart anomalies (20% tetralogy of Fallot). Cleft palate is present in 9% of cases and 36% have structural urinary tract abnormalities. Karyotyping is indicated and the microdeletion easily confirmed using fluorescent in-situ hybridization (FISH).

- If the diagnosis is made antenatally, fetal echocardiography and a detailed anomaly scan should be performed to look for common associated anomalies. Neonatal calcium levels should be monitored. Feeding problems are common and referral to a plastic surgeon and feeding specialist necessary.
- If one parent carries the 22q11 deletion, the recurrence risk is 50%. If neither parent carries the deletion, the risk of recurrence is very small (<1%).

Klinefelter syndrome (47 XXY)
- Klinefelter syndrome is the most common sex chromosome disorder affecting 1 in 660 males. Increasing maternal age is a risk factor.
- The diagnosis is usually made incidentally following a prenatal diagnostic procedure. There are no reliable ultrasound findings to make/ suggest the diagnosis non-invasively.
- Males enter puberty normally but soon develop hypergonadotrophic hypogonadism with low testosterone levels. The testis involutes and infertility results. The IQ can vary widely, but many affected individuals have some degree of intellectual impairment.
- The recurrence risk is low (<1%). There is an increased risk of sex chromosome aneuploidy and trisomy 21 to the offspring of affected males (in the rare event of successful conception) and prenatal diagnosis is advisable.

Genetic syndromes

Beckwith–Widemann syndrome (BWS)
- BWS is a somatic overgrowth and cancer predisposition syndrome with an incidence of 1 in 13 700 individuals. Males and females are equally affected. The phenotypic spectrum of this disorder also includes certain types of hemihypertrophy.
- 85% of cases are sporadic. 10%–15% of cases of BWS are part of autosomal dominant pedigrees demonstrating preferential maternal transmission. The overall risk of cancer in children is 7.5% with the majority being embryonal (hepatoblastoma, Wilms). Most tumors present by the age of 8 years.
- BWS is a complex, multigenic disorder caused by alterations in growth regulatory genes on chromosome 11p15. A number of imprinted genes (*IGF2, H19, CDKN1C, LIT1*) involved in growth may be affected.
- Approximately 60% of patients carry an epigenetic error at one of the two imprinting centers (*DMR1* and *DMR2*) on 11p15. The next largest category is paternal uniparental disomy (20%). Chromosomal abnormalities are relatively rare and include paternal duplications (<1%) and inversions/translocations (<1%). Mutations in the gene *CDKN1C* are responsible for about 10% of cases.
- In 10%–15% of individuals with BWS, the etiology is unknown.
- There is a significant correlation between uniparental disomy (UPD) and hemihypertrophy.

1

- The recurrence risk due to paternal UPD is very low. If BWS is caused by 11p15 chromosome translocations/inversions/duplications, the recurrence risks may be as high as 50%. Recurrence risk may be up to 50% if either parent is affected.
- If karyotype and UPD analysis are normal and, in the absence of any family history, the risk of recurrence is approximately 5%.

Duchenne and Becker muscular dystrophy

- Duchenne muscular dystrophy (DMD) affects 1 in 3500 male births. It is the most common and severe form of childhood muscular dystrophy. The mean age of loss of mobility is 9 years followed by death in the late teens or early 20s.
- Becker muscular dystrophy (BMD) is clinically similar to Duchenne but with milder symptoms. The average age of onset is 11 years with late (40–50 years) loss of the ability to walk.
- Both are X-linked recessive disorders caused by mutations in the dystrophin gene. 60%–65% of DMD is caused by large out-of-frame mutations. 5% of cases are caused by exon duplication with the remaining cases caused by nonsense or frameshift mutations that result in chain termination.
- 30% of affected individuals will have mild developmental delay that is usually not progressive. The cause of death is usually respiratory insufficiency and cardiomyopathy. There is also a high risk of developing scoliosis.
- BMD is caused by in-frame mutations in the dystrophin gene that cause reduced amounts of dystrophin being produced.
- 20% of female carriers of DMD have evidence of cardiac involvement and may also have proximal muscle weakness. BMD carriers are much less frequently and severely affected.
- A carrier female is at 25% risk of producing an affected son and a carrier daughter, respectively. Penetrance is complete in affected males.
- Prenatal diagnosis is available to carriers of a known dystrophin mutation. The method of choice is a chorionic villous sample at 11–13 weeks' gestation.
- Even if the precise mutation has not been detected, linkage analysis may identify a "high risk X," which can be used in prenatal diagnosis.
- Prenatal diagnosis is offered to carrier women who are carrying male fetuses. Fetal sexing using free fetal DNA in maternal blood is now available.

Fragile X syndrome

- Fragile sites are gaps, constrictions, or breaks on metaphase chromosomes that arise when cells are exposed to a perturbation of the DNA replication process. Fragile sites are seen on all human chromosomes and are named according to the chromosome band they are observed in.
- Fragile X syndrome is the most common form of inherited mental retardation with an incidence of 1 in 4000–6000 males. It is characterized

1

by a constellation of clinical manifestations, including mild to severe mental retardation, hyperactivity, and autism.

- The fragile site FRAXA is expressed in fragile X syndrome. The causative mutation is a (CGG) expansion of the 5'-untranslated region of the X-linked *FMR1* gene (Xq27.3). The expansion mutation leads to the hypermethylation of the promoter region resulting in silencing of the gene, causing reduced expression of the Fragile X Mental Retardation Protein (FMRP).
- The *FMR1* CGG repeat is polymorphic in the general population, with a normal range of 6–53 repeats. Alleles having between 55 and 200 CGG repeats are called premutations and generate *FMR1* mRNA and FMRP protein. Repeats in the premutation range are unstable in females and can expand further during oogenesis and postzygotic mitosis. The premutation frequency in the general population is approximately 1 in 259 in females and 1 in 813 in males.
- Affected individuals and full mutation carrier females have in excess of 200 CGG repeats.
- The fragile site FRAXE is less common with an incidence of 1 in 23 000 males. It is caused by a different repeat (GCC) in the *FMR2* gene on Xq28. Affected males have less severe disease.
- In females with a premutation, expansion of the repeat may not occur in every pregnancy although a massive expansion into the affected range is always a possibility. Males with the premutation will pass it on to all their daughters but none of their sons. The repeat size tends to remain stable.
- Prenatal diagnosis is possible using chorionic villi. A larger sample is usually required.

Myotonic dystrophy
- This is an autosomal dominant neuromuscular condition with a prevalence of 1:8000.
- Two genetic loci (DM1 on chromosome 19 and DM2 on chromosome 3) are associated with the myotonic dystrophy phenotype. The mutation responsible for DM1 is a CTG expansion located in the 3'-untranslated region of the dystrophia myotonica–protein kinase gene (DMPK), whereas DM2 is linked to CCTG expansion in intron 1 of the zinc finger protein gene ZNF9.
- Affected individuals have expansion repeats of >50. Affected females (>1000 repeats) who are symptomatic are at risk of a congenitally affected infant.
- Polyhydramnios is a common finding and the affected baby is frequently very floppy with diaphragmatic hypoplasia. Neonatal mortality may be as high as 20%. Preterm labor and postpartum hemorrhage are additional risks.
- The risk of having a child with features of myotonic dystrophy depends on the sex of the transmitting parent and degree of clinical severity. Mothers who are asymptomatic with a small repeat (<80) tend not to have affected babies. The mutation is transmitted in a relatively stable fashion.

GENETICS

- If the mother has neuromuscular involvement and a moderate expansion (200–500 repeats) with no previous affected child, the risk of congenital disease is 20%–30%. If there has been a previously affected child, the risk increases to 40%–50%.
- The risk of congenital myotonic dystrophy due to transmission from an affected father is very small.
- Affected families are at risk of anticipation with a tendency of increasing severity in subsequent generations.
- Prenatal diagnosis by CVS is possible although predicting the prognosis is more difficult. Most affected babies will have >1000 repeats.

Noonan syndrome
- This is an autosomal dominant condition with an incidence of 1 in 2500. It is caused by a mutation in the *PTPN11* gene on chromosome 12q. A family history is present in half of the cases. Some cases may occur as a result of new mutations.
- Affected fetuses can manifest nuchal edema and lymphatic abnormalities. Pulmonary stenosis may be present. Polyhydramnios may also be a feature of the pregnancy.
- Prenatal diagnosis for the *PTPN11* gene mutation is possible.

Tuberous sclerosis
- Tuberous sclerosis is a dominantly inherited disease of high penetrance, characterized by the presence of hamartomata in multiple organ systems, developmental delay, skin lesions, and seizures. Renal angiomyolipomata, cysts, and carcinoma are also features of the disease.
- The condition is highly penetrant but variable in its clinical manifestation.
- 60% of cases arise as new mutations. The condition is caused by mutations in the *TSC1* gene on chromosome 9q and *TSC2* gene on chromosome 16p.
- Cardiac rhabdomyomas identified on prenatal ultrasound are a well-recognized feature of congenital tuberous sclerosis. The risk of the baby being affected is >50%.
- An affected parent has a 50% risk of transmitting the mutant gene. If neither parent is affected, the risk is 2% due to germline mosaicism.
- Prenatal diagnosis is possible if the mutation is known.

ANEUPLOIDY SCREENING

- Chromosome abnormalities occur in 0.1%–0.2% of all live births with Down syndrome being the most clinically significant, due to the high incidence of mental handicap and associated structural malformations.
- Screening is the identification of a subset of the screened population, whose increased risk is high enough to warrant a diagnostic test. Screening is generally used for conditions that are clinically significant and prevalent in the population.
- Maternal age is a poor screening criterion, since the majority of children with Down syndrome are born to women younger than 35 years of age.
- The optimal screening test has a low false-positive rate, which will vary according to the maternal age of the population being screened. A false-positive rate of <5% is considered desirable. An ideal screening test should have a high detection rate (sensitivity) for the condition. However, as the detection rate increases, the false-positive rate will also rise, thereby increasing the number of women who will screen positive and require a diagnostic test.
- Screening for aneuploidy or fetal structural anomalies allows parents several choices after a definitive diagnosis is made. This may include preparation for the birth of a child with special needs as well as a management plan for the diagnosis and possible treatment of the condition. In some cases termination of pregnancy may be an option.
- Down syndrome is the most common genetic cause of mental retardation. It is associated with a number of structural malformations (usually cardiac) of varying severity and universal developmental delay. The risk increases with advancing maternal age.
- Down syndrome pregnancies are associated with decreased levels of maternal serum alphafetoprotein (AFP) and unconjugated estriol (uE3) and elevated levels of human chorionic gonadotropin (hCG) (either intact human chorionic gonadotropin or the free beta subunit).
- The median levels of the various hormones in Down syndrome pregnancies in the second trimester are as follows: hCG 2.06 multiples of the median (MoM), AFP 0.72 MoM, Inhibin A 1.79 MoM and unconjugated estriol 0.64 MoM.

First trimester screening

- Nuchal translucency (NT) by itself has an approximately 60% detection rate for Down syndrome with a 5% false-positive rate. However, this method has been superseded by the combined test which incorporates the use of pregnancy associated plasma protein A (PAPP-A) and hCG levels.
- Increased NT is also associated with other chromosomal abnormalities (including trisomy 18 and trisomy 13, Turner's syndrome, and triploidy), genetic disorders and fetal structural anomalies, particularly congenital heart defects.

2

- Two large, first and second trimester comparison studies: Serum, Urine, Ultrasound Study (SURUSS) in the UK, with more than 48 000 pregnancies, and First and Second Trimester Evaluation of Risk (FASTER) in the USA, with more than 36 000 pregnancies, had an 86% and 85% Down syndrome detection rate. The false-positive rate was approximately 5%. Together with two other large studies (BUN) (Blood, Ultrasound and Nuchal) study (USA) and the OSCAR (One stop clinic to assess risk) study (UK), the average detection rate for first trimester screening using the combined test is approximately 85% with a 5% false-positive rate.
- Median first trimester levels of PAPP-A and free beta hCG in Down syndrome pregnancies are 0.45 MoM and 1.79 MoM, respectively.

Second trimester screening

Serum screening

- This involves calculating a risk based on the maternal age and a blood sample taken between 15 and 22 weeks' gestation. Various screening tests are available: double test (AFP and hCG), triple test (AFP, hCG, and uE3) and quadruple test (AFP, hCG, uE3, and inhibin-A).
- The detection rates vary from 66% for the double test, 77% for the triple test to >80% for the quadruple test.
- Currently, only the combined, serum integrated, full integrated and the sequential integrated incorporate first trimester nuchal translucency measurement as a component of the test (Table 2.1).
- Integrated screening is used to calculate a single adjusted risk of Down syndrome after both the first and second trimester tests have been completed and is associated with a higher rate of detection of trisomy 21 (94%–96% in the FASTER trial and 94% in the SURUSS trial, with rates varying according to gestational age) than either first or second trimester screening alone.
- A major criticism of the integrated (i.e. first and second trimester testing) approach is the withholding of results from the first test until the second blood test is performed. Non-compliance rates of up to 25% for the second sample have been reported in some studies.
- To minimize non-compliance rates, and improve patient choice, two sequential screening strategies: stepwise and contingent screening have been proposed.
- Stepwise testing involves releasing the results of the first trimester combined screening to the patient and, if the risk of aneuploidy is greater than a predetermined cut-off level, the patient is then offered the option of proceeding with a diagnostic test. If the risk is not raised, the patient proceeds with the second trimester test and receives a revised and final risk assessment based on the first and second trimester measurements.
- Contingent sequential screening stratifies women according to the initial adjusted risk of Down syndrome. Only women with an intermediate risk would undergo the second trimester screening.

Table 2.1 *Different first and second trimester screening tests*

Test	Quadruple test	Combined test	Serum integrated	Full integrated	Sequential integrated
Components	AFP, uE3, hCG, inhibin-A	NT, PAPP-A, hCG	PAPP-A (first trimester), hCG, uE3, AFP, inhibin-A (second trimester)	NT and PAPP-A (first trimester), hCG, uE3, AFP, inhibin-A (second trimester)	NT and PAPP-A (first trimester), hCG, uE3, AFP, inhibin-A (second trimester)
Detection rate	80%–85%	85%–90%	85%–90%	85%–90%	85%–90%
False positive rate	5%–8%	4%–6%	4%–6%	1%–2%	1.5%–2.5%
Gestation performed	15–22 weeks (second trimester)	11.0–13.6 weeks (first trimester)	10.3–13.6 weeks and 15–22 weeks (first and second trimester)	10.3–13.6 weeks and 15–22 weeks (first and second trimester)	10.3–13.6 weeks and 15–22 weeks (first and second trimester)

2

Statistical modeling with the use of data from the FASTER trial gave detection rates of 91%–92% with false-positive rates of 4%–5%. With this approach, only 23% of women would require second trimester screening. Further research is needed to determine the most effective method of sequential screening and to compare it with other screening programs.

- By selecting a very high-risk cut-off for the first trimester portion of the stepwise and contingent approaches, the overall detection rate of these integrated test variants is kept high and the overall false-positive rate is kept low.

Soft markers of aneuploidy

- Studies have shown that second trimester ultrasonographic examination can identify 50%–75% of fetuses with Down syndrome, with false-positive rates of 4%–15%.
- Soft markers will be found in up to 15% of otherwise normal mid trimester pregnancies. When isolated, second trimester ultrasound markers such as choroid plexus cysts (Fig. 2.1), echogenic intracardiac focus (Fig. 2.2), echogenic bowel (EB) (Fig. 2.3), renal pelvis dilatation (Fig. 2.4), cerebral ventriculomegaly (Fig. 2.5), talipes (Fig. 2.6), shortened humerus, and shortened femur are not specific enough in either confirming or excluding Down syndrome (Table 2.2).
- Only a thickened nuchal fold (NF) (Fig. 2.7) **may** be useful in distinguishing between unaffected and affected fetuses. If a NF thickening is identified, the risk of Down syndrome is increased by approxi-mately 17×.
- The vast majority (>99%) of fetuses with an isolated ultrasound marker will, however, be unaffected. If ultrasound "soft" markers are used as an indicator for invasive testing, many unaffected fetuses may be lost as a complication of the procedure.

Second trimester hypoplastic nasal bone

- This is the latest described soft marker. The nasal bone in the second trimester is measured in a mid sagittal (profile) image and may be described as normal, absent, or hypoplastic (less than 2.5 mm). Approximately 0.5%–1.2% of normal fetuses and 43%–62% of trisomy 21 fetuses have an absent or hypoplastic nasal bone between 15 and 22 weeks. An absent nasal bone has been estimated to have a likelihood ratio of 83× the background rate, making this one of the most promising new markers.

Nuchal fold

- Although a thickened NF has been associated with a greatly increased risk of trisomy 21, it is an uncommon finding in both Down syndrome

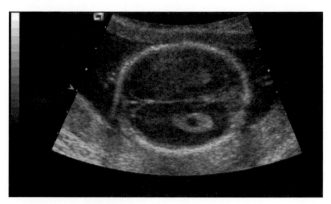

Fig. 2.1. Choroid plexus cyst.

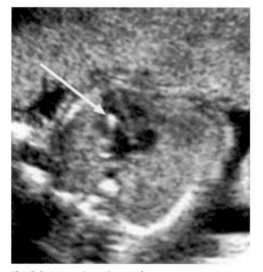

Fig. 2.2. Intracardiac echogenic focus.

and normal fetuses. It is even more uncommon in fetuses that have had a thin nuchal translucency measured previously. If this is the case, in addition to aneuploidy, alternative causes should be considered. It may reflect an early feature of fetal hydrops or cystic hygroma.

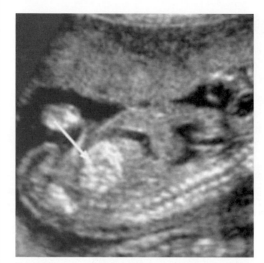

Fig. 2.3. Hyperechogenic bowel.

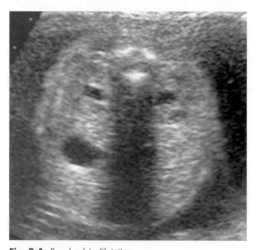

Fig. 2.4. Renal pelvis dilatation.

2

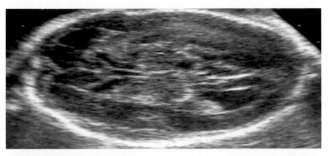

Fig. 2.5. Mild ventriculomegaly.

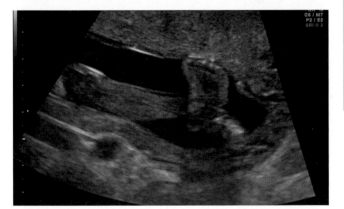

Fig. 2.6. Talipes.

Renal pelvis dilatation

- Approximately 17% of fetuses with trisomy 21 will have renal pelvic dilatation, although as an isolated abnormality it is a very uncommon finding in aneuploidy. The meta-analysis by Smith–Bindman in 2001 confirmed the lack of significance of this finding. Renal pelvis dilatation can be associated with a variety of urinary tract abnormalities and these babies should be reviewed later in pregnancy and after birth.

Echogenic bowel

- This is generally a rare finding (<1%) in normal fetuses compared with trisomy 21 fetuses (15%). EB is usually described as being at

Table 2.2 *Accuracy measures for each soft marker when identified as an isolated abnormality*

Marker	Sensitivity (95% CI)	Specificity (95% CI)	Positive LR (95% CI)	Negative LR (95% CI)	Women at average risk of a fetus with Down syndrome			Women at high risk of a fetus with Down syndrome		
					PPV	Number needed to screen	Fetal losses per case diagnosed	PPV	Fetal losses per case diagnosed	Number needed to screen
Thickened nuchal fold	0.04 (0.02–0.10)	0.99 (0.99–0.99)	17 (8–38)	0.97 (0.94–1.00)	0.024	15 893	0.6	0.053	0.2	6818
Choroid plexus cyst	0.01 (0–0.03)	0.99 (0.97–1.00)	1.00 (0.12–9.4)	1.00 (0.97–1.00)	0.002	87 413	4.3	0.003	1.8	37 500
Femur length	0.16 (0.05–0.40)	0.96 (0.94–0.98)	2.7 (1.2–6.0)	0.87 (0.75–1.00)	0.004	4454	1.2	0.009	0.5	1911
Humerus length	0.09 (0–0.60)	0.97 (0.91–0.99)	7.5 (4.7–12)	0.87 (0.67–1.1)	0.011	8038	1.9	0.024	0.8	3448
Echogenic bowel	0.04 (0.01–0.24)	0.99 (0.97–1.00)	6.1 (3.0–12.6)	1.00 (0.98–1.00)	0.009	19 425	1.0	0.020	0.4	8333
Echogenic intracardiac focus	0.11 (0.06–0.18)	0.96 (0.94–0.97)	2.8 (1.5–5.5)	0.95 (0.89–1.00)	0.004	6536	2.0	0.009	0.8	2804
Renal pyelectasis	0.02 (0.01–0.06)	0.99 (0.98–1.00)	1.9 (0.7–5.1)	1.00 (1.00–1.00)	0.003	30 404	2.6	0.006	1.1	13 043

The positive predictive value (PPV), fetal losses per case of Down syndrome diagnosed, and the number of women who would need to be screened for each case of Down syndrome identified were calculated for two hypothetical cohorts: women at average risk of carrying a fetus with Down syndrome, defined as the population risk (1:700), and those at high risk of carrying a fetus with Down syndrome, defined as the mid trimester risk in a 35-year-old woman (1:300). CI indicates confidence interval; and LR, likelihood ratio.

(Adapted from Smith-Bindman et al. *JAMA* 2001.)

2

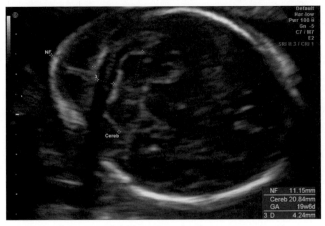

Fig. 2.7. Mid trimester nuchal edema. See color plate section.

least as bright as bone. Newer ultrasound machines, particularly with the harmonics function, may give a brighter appearance to the bowel and lead to more false-positives. A third of fetuses with true echogenic bowel will have some underlying pathology. First trimester bleeding, fetal infections, and cystic fibrosis are other possible causes. The parents should be counseled about this risk and offered parental testing for cystic fibrosis carrier status.

Shortened long bones

- Shortened humerus and femur have both been associated with an increased risk of chromosomal abnormalities. Many studies suggest the humerus is a more reliable marker for Down syndrome than the femur. Different authors have used various definitions of shortened long bones, including the observed length divided by expected length, or long bones below the 2.5th centile from standard charts. Other causes of shortened long bones include skeletal dysplasia or early-onset intrauterine growth restriction. Serial scans may be necessary to monitor fetal growth.

INVASIVE PROCEDURES

- There are many diagnostic and therapeutic invasive fetal procedures that can be performed during pregnancy. Some are technically simple with minimal risks, whilst others are lengthy complex procedures with much higher complication rates.
- All patients should be counseled at length about the proposed procedures and given written information before consent is obtained.
- All complex procedures should be performed in a tertiary center where comprehensive fetal medicine, imaging, and pediatric facilities exist. Referral to these centers should take place as early as possible, so that all options (including termination of pregnancy) can be discussed with the patient.
- Amniocentesis and CVS do not require prophylactic antibiotics. All other complex procedures should be covered and consideration also given for prophylactic tocolytics (e.g. indomethacin, progesterone, nifedipine).
- Maximum information should be obtained from any fetal sample collected. If a genetic syndrome is suspected, the cytogenetics laboratory should be asked to extract and store DNA from the sample so that any future gene tests are possible.
- Anti-D immunoglobulin prophylaxis should be administered to RhD negative women.

Amniocentesis

- One of the most commonly performed prenatal diagnostic procedures. Suitable for a variety of indications: karyotyping, detect evidence of intrauterine infection, evaluating fetal lung maturity (lecithin/sphingomyelin ratio), etc.
- Only active maternal HIV infection is an absolute contraindication to the procedure.
- Generally performed beyond 15 weeks under continuous ultrasound guidance (Fig. 3.1). Amniocentesis performed before 15 completed weeks of gestation is referred to as early.
- Higher rates of successful taps and lower rates of blood stained samples is achieved when it is performed under direct ultrasound control with continuous needle tip visualization.
- Whenever possible, the placenta should be avoided. However, a transplacental approach is not contraindicated if it provides easy access to a pool of amniotic fluid, but care should be taken to avoid the cord insertion. The outer needle diameter should not be wider than 20-gauge (0.9 mm).
- One milliliter of amniotic fluid is aspirated for every week of gestation up to a maximum of 20–22 ml. This is sufficient for most investigations.

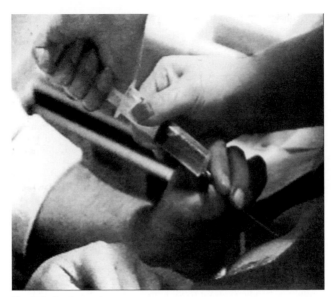

Fig. 3.1. Amniocentesis.

- The only large-scale prospective randomized study evaluating loss rates after mid trimester amniocentesis showed a 1% greater pregnancy loss rate in patients randomly assigned to undergo amniocentesis compared with those assigned to undergo ultrasound surveillance alone. More recent data suggest that the loss rate following amniocentesis is approximately 0.5%–0.6%.
- The recent First And Second Trimester Evaluation of Risk for aneuploidy (FASTER) study showed that the spontaneous fetal loss rate <24 weeks in the study group was 1.0% and was not statistically different from the background 0.94% rate seen in the control group. The procedure-related loss rate after amniocentesis was **0.06%** (1.0% minus the background rate of 0.94%). This equates to an amniocentesis procedure-related loss risk of approximately 1 in 1600 and is substantially lower than the traditionally quoted risk of 1 in 200.
- Early (11–13 weeks) compared with mid trimester amniocentesis is associated with a 3-fold increase in procedure loss rates (2.6% versus 0.8%) and a 13-fold increase in the incidence of talipes (1.3% versus 0.1%), 8-fold culture failure rate (1.7% versus 0.2%) and a doubling of the incidence of amniotic fluid leakage (3.5% versus 1.7%).
- CVS is the safer choice for patients desiring invasive prenatal diagnosis before 13 completed weeks. At 14 weeks, the data are not definitive in either direction.

- In equally experienced hands, CVS and second trimester amniocentesis have comparable safety outcomes.
- Both fluorescent in situ hybridization (FISH) and polymerase chain reaction (PCR) techniques can be used to exclude aneuploidy of selected chromosomes (usually chromosomes 13, 18, and 21).
- Full karyotype results generally take 14 days because of the need to grow the amniocytes in culture before metaphase analysis of the chromosomes.
- Third trimester amniocentesis does not appear to be associated with significant risk of emergency delivery. Compared with mid trimester procedures, complications including multiple attempts and blood-stained fluid are more common. Culture failure rates are also higher (9.7%), but PCR results are almost always obtainable.
- Amniocentesis and CVS in multiple pregnancies should be performed only by a specialist who has the expertise to carry out selective termination of pregnancy in the event of a discordant result. Placental and fetal mapping are essential prior to the procedure.
- Written information and formal consent for any invasive procedure is mandatory. Current UK guidelines suggest that the following should be provided: national and local risks of the procedures, analysis (and subsequent storage) of the sample in the local cytogenetics laboratory, accuracy of the particular laboratory test being performed, culture failure rates, reporting time, method of communication of results, and indications for seeking medical advice following the test.
- Anti-D immunoglobulin prophylaxis should be given to all RhD-negative women.

Chorionic villous sampling

- CVS is usually performed between 10 and 13 weeks of gestation and involves aspiration of placental tissue for analysis. CVS can be performed using either percutaneous transabdominal or the transcervical approach. Transabdominal CVS can be performed at gestations greater than 13 weeks.
- Rapid aneuploidy results for chromosomes 13, 18, and 21 are possible using FISH or PCR methods. The full karyotype generally takes 14 days.
- Chorionic villus samples typically contain a mixture of placental villi and maternally derived decidua (Figs. 3.2 and 3.3), which needs to be cleaned and separated before cytogenetic analysis can be carried out.
- Maternal cells may occasionally remain and grow in culture. As a result, two cell lines, one fetal and the other maternal, may be identified. Occasionally, the maternal cell line may completely overgrow the culture, leading to diagnostic errors.
- The second source of potential error is confined placental mosaicism (CPM), which occurs in approximately 1 in 200 cases.
- Mosaicism can occur through two possible mechanisms: trisomy (meiotic) rescue of a trisomic conceptus or mitotic postzygotic errors, producing a mosaic morula or blastocyst. Trisomy rescue may result in UPD.

3

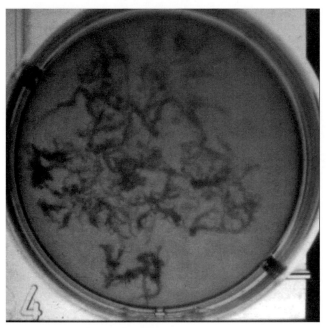

Fig. 3.2. CVS sample. See color plate section.

INVASIVE PROCEDURES

- Confined placental mosaicism unassociated with UPD has been shown to alter placental function and lead to fetal growth restriction or perinatal death. This is seen classically in CPM for chromosome 16, which leads to severe intrauterine growth restriction, prematurity, or perinatal death, with less than 35% of pregnancies resulting in normal, appropriate-for-gestational-age, full-term infants.
- The role of CVS in dichorionic placentae remains controversial because of a relatively high risk of cross contamination of chorionic tissue leading to false positive or false negative results. Such procedures should be performed by experienced operators only in exceptional circumstances after detailed counseling.
- CVS has a miscarriage risk of 2%–3% over that of mid trimester amniocentesis. However, as with any procedure, the risks are largely operator dependent and many experienced practitioners have similar low miscarriage rates for both procedures.
- Early CVS (before 9 weeks) might cause limb and other defects by transient fetal hypoperfusion and vasospastic phenomena secondary to vascular disruption to the placental circulation. The risk may be as high as 1%–2%.

3

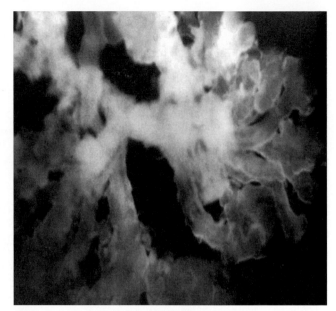

Fig. 3.3. Chorionic villi. See color plate section.

- There is no increase in risk of limb reduction defects if CVS is done after 11 weeks' gestation.
- Similar consent and counseling procedures (as for amniocentesis) should be followed.
- Anti-D immunoglobulin prophylaxis should be given to all RhD-negative women.

Fetal blood sampling and intrauterine transfusion

- Fetal blood sampling can be performed for a variety of reasons (karyotyping, ascertaining fetal acid–base status, transfusion of blood or platelets, direct fetal therapy for fetal arrhythmias, etc).
- The two common sites used are the intrahepatic vein (Fig. 3.4) or the umbilical vein at the placental cord insertion site. Sampling from a free loop is also possible but is technically more challenging and has higher complication rates. The intrahepatic approach has lower complication rates compared with the umbilical cord.
- The procedure is performed under aseptic conditions and continuous ultrasound guidance. Prophylactic maternal antibiotics should be administered.

3

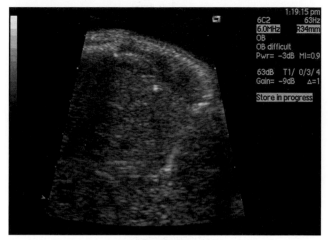

Fig. 3.4. Fetal blood sampling from the hepatic vein.

INVASIVE PROCEDURES

- Fetal paralysis may be used, depending on operator preference. In most cases this is not necessary. There is some evidence that fetal paralysis may decrease the incidence of fetal distress.
- A recent large review of fetal blood sampling and intrauterine transfusion showed an overall obstetric complication rate of 17%. However, the procedure-related complication rate was approximately 3% per procedure. The procedure-related perinatal loss rate was 1.6% per procedure. Complications included rupture of membranes and preterm delivery, infection, emergency cesarean section, and perinatal death. Emergency cesarean section and perinatal death were the commonest complications.
- Preterm rupture of membranes/preterm delivery are relatively uncommon complications, with rates as low as 0.1% being reported.
- Although the incidence of intrauterine infection does not appear to be increased in women who do not receive prophylactic antibiotics compared with those who do, most centers do administer a single dose of pre-procedure antibiotics.
- Procedure-related fetal bradycardia requiring delivery is a serious complication of fetal blood sampling, particularly at very preterm gestations. In a low-risk population the risk is approximately 1.5%–3% but, if the fetus is hydropic, the risk is substantially increased (20%).
- Intrauterine transfusion has a mean procedure-related loss rate of 2.0% per procedure.
- Procedure-related fetal distress is usually due to either local cord complications (hematoma and arterial spasm) or to excessive bleeding followed by fetal exsanguination.

3

- Bleeding from the puncture site has been reported more frequently in hydropic fetuses because of thrombocytopenia. Some practitioners perform concomitant administration of platelets to minimize this risk. In the majority of cases this is not necessary.
- Arterial puncture is a well-known risk factor for bradycardia and fetal distress. The most plausible explanation for complications after arterial puncture is local vasospasm, although thrombosis and artery regression have been described. If arterial puncture occurs inadvertently, the procedure should be stopped because of the risk of fetal distress (17%–30%) and death (10%).
- Because of the technical difficulties in performing fetal blood sampling/intrauterine transfusion prior to 20 weeks, the complication rates are higher. A procedure related loss rate of 5%–6% is common.
- At viable gestations the patient must be counseled about the potential for emergency delivery if a complication arises. This has significant implications, particularly if the fetus is hydropic or if the procedure is done at very preterm gestations when ex-utero complications of prematurity may be very serious.

Feticide

- The current guidelines from the Royal College of Obstetricians and Gynecologists state that, for all terminations at gestational age of more than 21 weeks and 6 days, *the method chosen should ensure that the fetus is born dead*.
- Feticide should be undertaken by an appropriately trained practitioner. Intracardiac potassium chloride is the recommended method and the dose chosen should ensure that fetal asystole has been achieved.
- The commonest fetal indication for feticide in a recent large series was aneuploidy followed by brain malformations. Maternal indications included severe pre-eclampsia, heart disease, and psychiatric disorders.
- 1% of all terminations in the UK is by direct fetal injection of a lethal agent (e.g. potassium chloride).
- The procedure should be performed under aseptic conditions with continuous ultrasound control. The needle should be introduced into the left ventricle and the tip clearly seen. After aspirating 1 ml of fetal blood to confirm correct needle placement potassium chloride is injected. The average amount of potassium chloride required to achieve asystole is approximately 5 ml, but this will depend on the gestation of the fetus.
- Injection into the umbilical cord can also be performed, although this may be associated with longer procedure times and the need to perform direct intra-cardiac injection in a proportion of cases. A few cases of failed feticide with the birth of a live baby have also been reported.
- Inadvertent maternal injection has never been reported. Correct needle placement is essential before the potassium chloride is injected.

3

- It is good practice to discuss all cases in a multidisciplinary forum before a final decision regarding the offer of late termination is made.
- Ideally, if feticide is required in a multiple pregnancy following karyotyping, the fetal medicine specialist who initially performed the amniocentesis should also be the practitioner performing the feticide. Careful mapping of the placenta and fetuses is required to ensure that the correct fetus is identified before termination.

Statutory registration requirements in the UK
- When a fetus is born before the 24 + 0 weeks of gestation and did not breathe or show signs of life (detectable heart rate), there is no provision for the event to be registered. However, the doctor or midwife who attended the delivery will need to issue a certificate or letter for the funeral director, cemetery, or crematorium stating that the baby was born before the legal age of viability and showed no signs of life to allow a funeral to proceed, if that is the parents' wish.
- When a child is born after 24 + 0 weeks but did not breathe or show any sign of life, it is classified as a *stillbirth*. Stillbirths require registration within 3 months. In the event of a child being born which shows signs of life but subsequently dies, both the birth and death need to be registered, irrespective of the gestation period of the child.
- In cases where there are *any signs of life* the baby must been seen by a medical practitioner and that practitioner must sign the death certificate (otherwise it becomes a Coroner's case). Fetuses known to have died in utero before 24 + 0 weeks, but born after this gestational threshold, do not require registration. This is important in cases of multiple pregnancy, where one or more fetuses are known to have died in utero, either spontaneously or following fetal reduction.

Fetal shunts

- Pleuro-amniotic and vesico-amniotic shunts (Fig. 3.5) are procedures performed in selected cases of fetal pulmonary effusion and an enlarged bladder secondary to lower urinary tract obstruction. Thoracic shunts can also be used to drain large pulmonary cysts that cause significant cardiac compression and hydrops.
- The rationale for pleuro-amniotic shunting is mainly to prevent pulmonary hypoplasia secondary to lung compression from a large pleural effusion or cyst. In some cases, hydrops due to cardiac compression can resolve once the chest is decompressed.
- Prophylactic antibiotics should be administered pre-procedure. Local anesthetic is required due to the size of the shunt introducers. The shunts should be inserted under continuous ultrasound guidance. Fetal paralysis is generally not required, although may be necessary in very selected cases.
- The risk of pre-labour rupture of membranes may be as high as 20%, and higher still if the fetus is hydropic or if polyhydramnios is present.

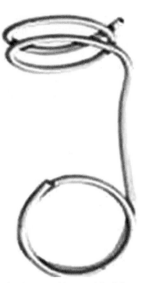

Fig. 3.5. Double pig-tail fetal shunt.

- Serial scans are necessary to check resolution of the pleural effusion, bladder decompression and decrease in hydronephrosis and improvement in hydrops.
- Fetal shunts can get easily obstructed from blood or vernix. The fetus can also pull the shunt out. Shunt migration is a known complication, especially with vesico-amniotic shunts, which can be pulled into an intra-abdominal or intravesical location particularly if inserted too high. Pleuro-amniotic shunts can migrate into the pleural cavity. If shunts migrate into an intra-fetal location, surgery may be required for their removal.
- Anterior abdominal wall defects (iatrogenic gastroschisis) have been reported secondary to vesico-amniotic shunt insertion. Direct fetal organ damage has also been reported.

Multifetal pregnancy reduction (MFPR)

- Multifetal pregnancy reduction is defined as a first trimester or early second trimester termination of one or more fetuses in a multifetal pregnancy, to improve the perinatal outcome of the remaining fetuses.
- There is an increasing incidence of triplets and higher-order multiples with artificial reproductive techniques. The risks of maternal and perinatal morbidity and mortality are directly related to the number of fetuses.

- Triplets fare worse than twins, both in terms of gestation and birth weight. They have a 10× greater risk of being extremely low birth weight (<1000 g), which in addition to prematurity is an additional risk factor for adverse perinatal outcome. The perinatal mortality rate for triplets is almost 30% and for quadruplets close to 45%.

- For triplets, the average gestational age at delivery is 33 weeks, with 25% delivering prior to 32 weeks and 8% prior to 28 weeks. Quadruplets deliver even earlier, with 45% delivering prior to 32 weeks and 14% prior to 28 weeks.

- In triplet and higher-order multiple pregnancy, it is critical that patients are counseled about the risks associated with the pregnancy and referred to a fetal medicine specialist for consideration of MFPR. Failure to do so is considered substandard care.

- Published data clearly indicate that the higher the plurality, the greater the prevalence of cerebral palsy. There is a significant exponential relationship with the number of fetuses.

- For MFPR procedures done transbdominally the overall loss rate is between 5% and 6%. There is a strong correlation between the loss rate and the starting number of fetuses. The majority of losses occur more than 4 weeks following the procedure.

- In most circumstances, the general recommendation is to reduce to twins, given the overall excellent outcomes of twins. However, given that the procedure-related loss rate for a 3 to 1 reduction is not substantially different from a 3 to 2 reduction (15% to 7% and 15% to 5%, respectively), the gestational age at delivery for the resulting singleton is higher, and the incidence of births <1500 g is 10% higher for twins than for singletons, there is good argument to at least consider this option in selected cases.

- MFPR is a procedure that must be undertaken in a tertiary fetal medicine unit with experience in invasive fetal procedures in multiple pregnancy. A full discussion should take place prior to the procedure, covering issues such as procedure-related complications, the risk–benefit ratio and the ethical implications in reducing fetuses when artificial reproductive techniques have been responsible for the conception in the first place.

- In general, the fetus furthest away from the cervix should be selected for reduction. Obviously abnormal fetuses (raised nuchal translucency, small crown rump length, abnormalities, etc.) would prompt reduction of the affected fetus.

- The presence of a monochorionic pair can significantly increase the risk of perinatal complications. In general, consideration should be given for reduction of the monochorionic pair. The use of radiofrequency and interstitial laser techniques now allow selective reduction of one of a monochorionic pair. The procedure-related risks are, however, higher.

4 CENTRAL NERVOUS SYSTEM ABNORMALITIES

Central nervous system (CNS)

- Development of the human CNS involves several complex steps including neural proliferation, neuroblast migration, and neuronal differentiation (Table 4.1). This is an extremely complex process influenced by both genetic and environmental factors.

Agenesis of the corpus callosum

- Agenesis of the corpus callosum (ACC) is a failure to develop the large bundle of fibers that connect the two cerebral hemispheres. It occurs in 1:4000 individuals and has been estimated to have an incidence of 4 per 1000 live births (Fig. 4.1).
- The corpus callosum develops between the 5th and 17th weeks of pregnancy, although a diagnosis of ACC should be made with caution prior to 20 weeks. The human corpus callosum contains approximately 190 million axons.
- Corpus callosum formation involves multiple steps, including correct midline patterning, formation of hemispheres, specification of commissural neurons, and axon guidance across the midline to their final target in the contralateral hemisphere. ACC can be either complete or partial (Figs. 4.2 and 4.3).
- ACC may occur in isolation, associated with aneuploidy, part of a genetic syndrome or in association with other brain malformations. Various teratogens (alcohol, anti-epileptic medication, and cocaine), environmental factors and viral infections (rubella) have also been associated with ACC.
- Mutations in the *ARX*, *L1CAM*, and *KCC3* genes have all been reported to be associated with ACC. In most individuals with ACC there is no clearly inherited cause or a recognized genetic syndrome, suggesting that ACC can be caused by sporadic genetic events. Alcohol may disrupt both the transcription and biochemical function of the *L1CAM* gene. The incidence of ACC in fetal alcohol syndrome is approximately 7%, with a very high incidence of other callosal abnormalities.
- Ultrasound features of ACC include increased separation of the frontal horns of the lateral ventricles. The posterior horns of the ventricles are more dilated ("teardrop" shape) and the third ventricle is more dilated and displaced superiorly. The interhemispheric fissure may also be more widened.
- If ACC is suspected, a careful search for both intracranial and extracranial anomalies is required. Karyotyping should be offered. Fetal MRI to assess the brain in greater detail should also be performed.
- The associated ventriculomegaly can be severe and may influence long-term outcome.

Table 4.1 *Milestones during human brain development*

Induction of neuroectoderm	3rd week
Neurulation	3rd–4th week
Formation of the prosencephalon and hemispheres	5th–10th week
Neuronal proliferation	10th–20th week
Neuronal migration	12th–24th week
Neuronal apoptosis	28th–40th week
Neurogenesis	15th–20th week onwards
Synaptogenesis and synaptic stabilisation	20th week onwards for many years
Glial formation	20th–24th weeks onwards
Myelination	36th–38th week onwards for 2–3 years
Angiogenesis	5th–10th weeks onwards for several years

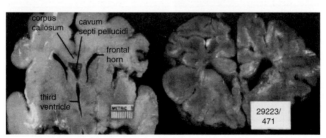

Fig. 4.1. Pathology specimen demonstrating normal brain and agenesis of the corpus callosum. See color plate section.

- Counseling by a pediatric neurologist is essential as the spectrum of potential problems is wide. Termination of pregnancy should be offered if the diagnosis is made prior to 24 weeks, or after this gestation if there is evidence of progressive ventriculomegaly, or the presence of additional abnormalities.
- The outcome for complete and partial ACC is conflicting, with the majority of studies showing no difference in behavioral and medical outcomes between the two.
- Most children with isolated ACC will have mild behavioral problems. Older data suggested that many individuals were normal; however, more sensitive assessment methods have revealed that deficits in

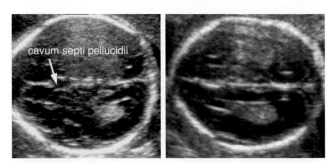

Fig. 4.2. Ultrasound images of normal brain (left) and agenesis of the corpus callosum (right).

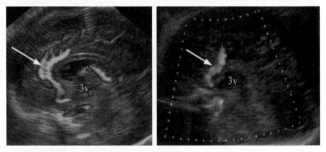

Fig. 4.3. Pericallosal artery. See color plate section.

higher-order cognition and social skills are present, even in the so-called "normal" individuals with ACC.

- Primary ACC has a surprisingly limited impact on general cognitive ability. Although the full-scale IQ scores can be lower than expected, based on family history, scores frequently remain within the average range. In as many as 60% of affected individuals, performance IQ and verbal IQ are significantly different.
- Patients with primary ACC also show marked difficulties with expressive language, have impaired social skills, and self-esteem. There are also many similarities with some neuropsychiatric disorders such as schizophrenia and autism.
- Recurrence risk for isolated ACC is estimated at 2%–3%.

Dandy–Walker malformation

- Dandy–Walker malformation (DWM) is the most common congenital malformation of the cerebellum with an incidence of 1 in 5000 births. Classic DWM is characterized by absence of the cerebellar vermis, accompanied dilatation of the fourth ventricle, and a posterior

4

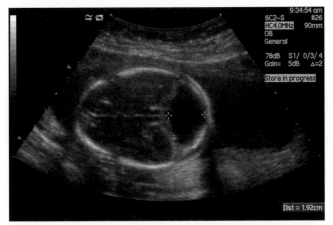

Fig. 4.4. Large posterior fossa cyst with hypoplastic cerebellum.

fossa cyst. The cerebellum itself may be hypoplastic (Figs. 4.4, 4.5, and 4.6).
- Some authors suggest that the Dandy–Walker complex be considered as a continuum of posterior fossa anomalies comprising the Dandy–Walker malformation, the Dandy–Walker variant, and mega cisterna magna. Cerebellar malformation appears to be the fundamental fault.
- In the Dandy–Walker variant, the posterior fossa is minimally enlarged; there is partial agenesis of the vermis, the fourth ventricle communicates with the arachnoid space, and no hydrocephalus is present. In mega cisterna magna the posterior fossa is prominent, secondary to an enlarged cisterna magna, but the vermis and fourth ventricle are normal.
- Dandy–Walker malformation can occur in association with a variety of genetic syndromes, chromosomal abnormalities, infections, or environmental teratogens.
- Associated CNS malformations are present in up to 68% of cases, the most common of which is agenesis or hypoplasia of the corpus callosum. Other CNS malformations include neuronal heterotopias, polymicrogyria, schizencephaly, occipital encephaloceles, and lumbosacral meningoceles.
- Extracranial malformations are found in about 30% of cases, particularly in familial syndromes, and include cleft lip and palate, cardiac malformations, urinary tract anomalies, and minor facial dysmorphisms.
- Mutations in *ZIC* genes (on chromosome 3) in humans have recently been implicated in a wide variety of congenital malformations, including Dandy–Walker malformation, holoprosencephaly, neural tube defects, and heterotaxy.

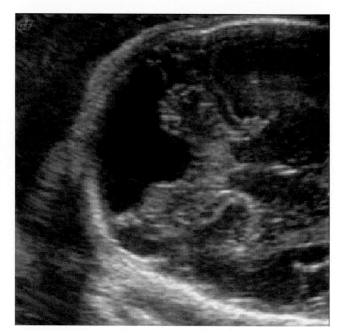

Fig. 4.5. Dandy–Walker malformation with agenesis of the vermis.

- When detected, additional structural anomalies need to be excluded. Karyotyping should be offered. In selected cases, particularly if Dandy–Walker variant is suspected, fetal MRI is extremely helpful.
- Termination of pregnancy is an option, regardless of gestation if a classic Dandy–Walker malformation is detected, because of the very poor long-term prognosis. The situation is more difficult with isolated Dandy–Walker variant, as many of these children may have a good long-term outcome. However, if the diagnosis is made prior to 24 weeks, or if there are additional anomalies, termination of pregnancy should be discussed. Counseling by a pediatric neurologist is essential.
- If a genetic syndrome is detected, genetic counseling should be arranged and, where appropriate, prenatal diagnosis offered.
- There is no fetal therapy and this abnormality does not influence the mode of delivery.
- The majority of children with isolated Dandy–Walker variant abnormality are free of major neurodevelopmental and functional disability. However, overall developmental, functional, and behavioral profiles are slightly poorer compared with normal infants. Problems

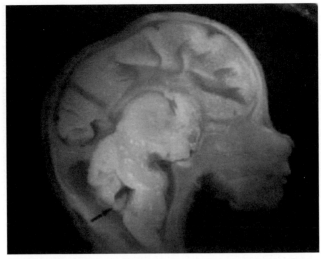

Fig. 4.6. Pathology specimen demonstrating cerebellar vermis hypoplasia. See color plate section.

include developmental delay in gross and fine motor skills and expressive language ability, which can result in functional difficulties in motor, social, and communication skills.

- The recurrence risk of non-syndromic DWM has been estimated to be approximately 1%–2%.

Holoprosencephaly

- Holoprosencephaly (HPE) is a spectrum of congenital malformations involving the brain and face and is characterized by impaired or incomplete midline division of the embryonic forebrain (prosencephalon). Holoprosencephaly has an incidence of 1 in 16 000 live births. Only 3% of fetuses with HPE survive to birth.

- Facial anomalies associated with HPE include cyclopia, ethmocephaly, cebocephaly, median cleft lip, and less severe facial manifestations (Fig. 4.7). Although midline facial defects occur in the majority (>80%) of cases, less severe facial dysmorphism (single central incisor and/or mild ocular hypotelorism) are associated with some mild forms of HPE.

- The first HPE gene identified in humans was the *Sonic Hedgehog* (*SHH*) gene located on chromosome 7. *SHH* mutations have been detected most frequently in HPE patients, and 17% of familial HPE cases and 3%–4% of sporadic HPE cases are known to have a *SHH* mutation. *ZIC2* gene (on chromosome 13) mutations are detected in 3%–4% cases of HPE. There are many other genes (*SIX3, TGIF, TDGF1, FAST1, PTCH, GLI2,* and *DHCR7*), which are associated with the development of HPE.

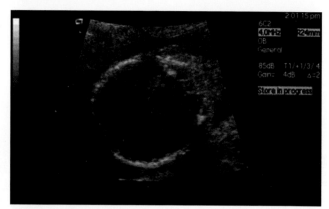

Fig. 4.7. Alobar holoprosencephaly with large single ventricle.

- Microdeletions in the four main HPE genes (*SHH*, *ZIC2*, *SIX3*, *TGIF*) are a common cause of prenatal HPE in euploid fetuses.
- Human HPE can be divided into two categories with different phenotypes: classic and middle interhemispheric (MIH).
- Classic HPE is divided into alobar, semilobar, and lobar subtypes on the basis of severity and the extent of hemispheric separation. Alobar is the most severe. Craniofacial involvement and forebrain midline defects are most severe. Abnormalities in the hypothalamus, pituitary gland, and basal ganglia are frequently seen in classic HPE.
- The MIH form selectively involves the middle interhemispheric region (the posterior frontal and parietal lobes in humans) and does not have significant craniofacial or ventral forebrain abnormalities.
- Alobar HPE is the most severe form. With complete division of the cerebral hemispheres with a single midline forebrain ventricle (monoventricle), which often communicates with a dorsal cyst. The interhemispheric fissure and corpus callosum are completely absent (Fig. 4.7).
- In semilobar HPE, there is a failure of separation of the anterior hemispheres, with some separation of the posterior hemispheres. The frontal horns of the lateral ventricle are absent, but posterior horns are present. The corpus callosum is absent anteriorly.
- In lobar HPE (the mildest form), the cerebral hemispheres are fairly well divided, with fusion of only the most rostral/ventral aspects.
- Approximately 40% of live births with HPE have a chromosomal anomaly and trisomy 13 accounts for over half of these cases. Of infants born with trisomy 13, 70% have holoprosencephaly. Aneuploidy confers a much worse prognosis, with only 2% surviving beyond 1 year.

- In addition to aneuploidy, several monogenic syndromes (Pallister–Hall, Meckel, Velocardiofacial and Smith–Lemli–Opitz) are associated with HPE.
- Multiple environmental factors have been implicated in the pathogenesis of HPE. Maternal diabetes, including gestational diabetes, is a well-established risk factor. A diabetic mother's risk of having a child with HPE is approximately 1%, a greater than 100-fold increase over the general population. Alcohol, anti-epileptic medication, retinoic acid, cigarette smoking, and congenital cytomegalovirus infection have all also been implicated.
- Once holoprosencephaly has been diagnosed, additional structural anomalies should be carefully searched for. In particular, facial malformations are common. There may be some degree of thalamic fusion. Differential diagnoses include ventriculomegaly, midline cerebral defects, hydrancephaly, arachnoid, or porencephalic cysts.
- Kayotyping must be offered. Termination of pregnancy should be discussed and offered.
- Alobar and most cases of semilobar HPE are not compatible with prolonged ex-utero survival. Lobar HPE or the middle interhemispheric anomalies can be associated with long-term survival and will need evaluation for endocrine abnormalities and/or craniofacial surgery.
- Genetic counseling is essential and prenatal diagnosis may be an option in selected cases. HPE due to euploid non-syndromic causes have an empiric recurrence risk of 6%.

Ventriculomegaly
- Ventriculomegaly is defined by a measurement of >10 mm of the atrium of the posterior or anterior horns of the lateral ventricles at any gestation. A measurement >15 mm is considered severe (Fig. 4.8).
- Ventriculomegaly can result from three processes. The first is obstruction to cerebrospinal fluid (CSF) flow or impaired absorption. The second is perturbations of cerebral development and may include either structural malformations (Dandy–Walker malformation) or aberrations of cortical development (neuronal migration syndromes). The third is destructive, and may result from vascular injury or infection.
- Routine ultrasound images of the fetal head should include those obtained at the level of the atrium of the lateral ventricle. Ventricular measurements should be obtained on a true transverse image of the fetal brain, as oblique views can over-estimate the ventricular dimensions. The third and fourth ventricles should also be measured if evident.
- Once detected, it is important to obtain a detailed history, especially of recent viral illness or maternal trauma, family genetic history, previous congenital abnormality, or fetal/neonatal thrombocytopenia.
- The fetal head and cerebellar shape and size, presence of intracranial calcifications, and extracerebral space (external hydrocephalus)

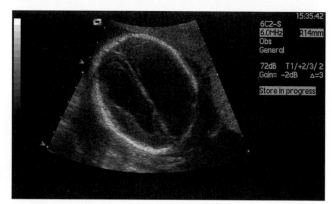

Fig. 4.8. Severe ventriculomegaly.

should be assessed. The brain should be carefully examined to exclude other associated cerebral malformations (e.g. Dandy–Walker malformation) which are frequently present. The spine must be examined in all three planes to exclude spina bifida.

- Limb movements should be assessed and the presence of talipes and/ or other signs of arthrogryposis should be excluded.
- Karyotyping should be offered (7%–15% risk of aneuploidy). Amniotic fluid can also be sent for viral PCR analysis. The risk of aneuploidy is higher if additional anomalies are present. If a small/ subtle spina bifida is suspected, amniotic fluid for AFP/AChE assays should be considered. Maternal blood for infection screening particularly toxoplasma/cytomegalovirus (CMV) and rubella should be performed. If severe ventriculomegaly is present in a male fetus an X-linked, cause should be considered and genetic testing for the *L1CAM* gene mutation performed.
- If the ventriculomegaly is associated with intracerebral hemorrhage, evidence of fetal alloimmune thrombocytopenia should be sought (antiplatelet antibodies/human platelet antigen (HPA) typing).
- Fetal MRI should be arranged and further review with a pediatric neurologist is essential, particularly if the prognosis is in doubt. Genetic counseling should be offered if appropriate.
- Neurodevelopmental outcome for mild isolated ventriculomegaly is variable and, in general, >85% will have a normal outcome or minimal delay. However, asymmetric bilateral ventriculomegaly may carry a worse prognosis with these children at a significant risk for behavioural abnormalities. Poor prognostic factors include co-existent cerebral anomalies, progression of the ventriculomegaly, and female sex.
- In severe ventriculomegaly, the outcome may still be variable but <30% of children will develop normally.

- Termination of pregnancy should be offered for severe ventriculo-megaly (>15 mm), aneuploidy, spina bifida, or other associated major malformations. Mode of delivery is on standard obstetric grounds. In the presence of severe macrocephaly, cesarean section or cephalocentesis may be required. Cephalocentesis is associated with a high incidence of procedural/intrapartum demise.
- Long-term follow-up is essential. If the ventriculomegaly is progressive or severe, neurosurgical intervention may be required after birth.

Neural tube defects

- Neurulation is the fundamental embryonic process that leads to the development of the neural tube, precursor of the brain, and spinal cord. Neurulation occurs through two distinct phases: primary neurulation (weeks 3–4) that leads to the formation of the brain and most of the spinal cord till the upper sacral level, followed by secondary neurulation (weeks 5–6) that creates the lowest portion of the spinal cord including most of the sacral and all the coccygeal regions.
- Closure of the neural tube involves apposition of the dorsal edges of the neural folds along the median plane, epithelial breakdown at contact sites accompanied by apoptosis and merger of the neuroepithelium.
- The development of the neural tube is a multi-step process strictly controlled by genes and modulated by a variety of environmental factors. It involves gene–gene, gene–environment and gene–nutrient interactions.
- Most neural tube defects are multifactorial in origin, with a genetic component that interacts with a number of environmental risk factors.
- The commonest forms of neural tube defects are referred to as open, where the involved neural tissues are exposed to the body surface. They include anencephaly, craniorachischisis, and myelomeningocele.
- Closed neural tube defects are categorized depending on the presence or absence of a lower back subcutaneous mass. Those with a mass include lipomyeloschisis, lipomyelomeningocele, meningocele, and myelocystocele. Closed defects without a mass include simple dysraphic states (intradural lipomas, diastematomyelia, teratoma, dermoid, epidermoid, tight filum terminale, persistent terminal ventricle, and dermal sinus) and complex dysraphic states (dorsal enteric fistula, neurenteric cysts, split cord malformations, caudal regression syndrome, and spinal segmental dysgenesis).
- 2%–16% of isolated open neural tube defects occur in association with aneuploidy or a single gene defect. If additional structural anomalies are present, the risk may be as high as 24%.
- Most cases of neural tube defects are multifactorial in origin. Anticonvulsant use, mutations in the *MTHFR* gene (methylene tetrahydrofolate reductase), maternal hyperthermia, obesity, diabetes mellitus, and a previous family history are all risk factors.

4

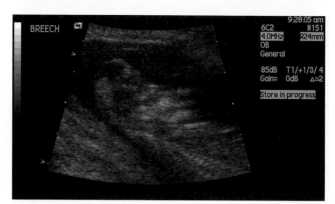

Fig. 4.9. First trimester fetus with anencephaly.

Anencephaly

- This is a lethal anomaly with a very high perinatal loss rate. Female fetuses are more commonly affected.
- The diagnosis is easily made on antenatal ultrasound. (Fig. 4.9) The facial bones and base of skull are generally well formed.
- Up to a third of cases may have additional structural malformations. There is an association with aneuploidy (trisomy 13 and 18), particularly if additional anomalies are present. Severe skull abnormalities can be associated with the amniotic band syndrome, although there should be evidence of other malformations (limb amputation, anterior abdominal wall defects).
- Polyhydramnios may be present in up to 50% of cases and is usually due to increased fluid and CSF loss from the exposed neural tissue and possibly from decreased fetal swallowing.
- Increased amniotic fluid in these pregnancies predisposes to preterm labour and placental abruption. Malpresentation and postpartum hemorrhage is also common.
- Termination of pregnancy should be offered once the diagnosis is made. Karyotyping should be offered. In pregnancies that continue regular monitoring for the development of polyhydramnios is necessary. The mode of delivery is decided on standard obstetric grounds.
- The parents should be counseled that, although this is a lethal condition, some babies may survive for several days and that only comfort care is appropriate.
- Although anencephalic fetuses are sometimes considered potential organ donors, in practice, this is difficult to achieve for several reasons – difficulty in diagnosing brain death, infection due to large area of exposed neural tissue, etc.
- Recurrence in any subsequent pregnancy can be significantly reduced by taking a high dose (4–5 mg) of folic acid periconceptually.

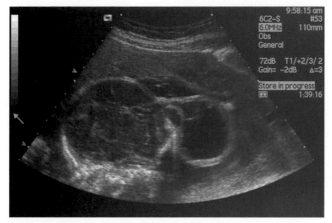

Fig. 4.10. Large posterior encephalocele containing brain tissue.

Encephalocele
- An encephalocele is a protrusion of part of the cranial contents through a defect in the skull. It may contain meninges (meningocele), meninges and brain (meningoencephalocele), or meninges, brain, and ventricle (meningoencephalocystocele).
- Encephaloceles are subdivided according to their anatomic location – frontal (sincipital), basal, occipital, convexity, and atretic encephaloceles.
- Frontal (sincipital) encephaloceles are further classified based on the fronto-ethmoidal internal defect through the foramen cecum, with more subdivisions into nasofrontal, nasoethmoidal and naso-orbital encephaloceles, depending on their facial exit anatomy. Facial clefts may be present and hypertelorism is a common accompaniment.
- Basal encephaloceles protrude through defects in the basal skull bones. They may be transethmoidal, sphenoethmoidal, spheno-maxillary, spheno-orbital, intrasphenoidal and transtemporal and transsphenoidal (often as part of the median cleft syndrome).
- Convexity encephaloceles occur anywhere (usually in the midline) on the vertex. Atretic encephaloceles are small skin-covered sub-scalp lesions often associated with other intracranial abnormalities.
- Occipital encephaloceles protrude through the occipital bone and occasionally through the foramen magnum or atlas. This is the commonest type of encephalocele in a Western population (Figs. 4.10 and 4.11).
- The diagnosis is usually made on antenatal ultrasound, which may show a cystic mass, a combined cystic–solid mass or a predominantly solid mass attached to the calvarium. A defect in the skull may sometimes be visible. 75% of encephaloceles are situated in the

4

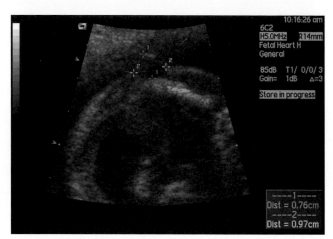

Fig. 4.11. Small occipital encephalocele.

occipital region and 15% in the frontal region and approximately 5% at the vertex.

- Up to 15% of cases may be associated with a concomitant neural tube defect. The head may be small (microcephaly present in 20%–50% of cases) because of the herniation of intracranial contents within the encephalocele.
- Differential diagnoses include cystic hygroma, lipomas of the scalp, teratomas or hemangiomas. Encephaloceles typically occur in the midline.
- Amniotic band syndrome can result in encephalocele formation particularly if occurring early in gestation. The defects are usually large, situated outside the midline and additional structural malformations are present.
- There is a significant association with genetic syndromes (Meckel–Gruber, Fraser, Roberts and Chemke's syndrome). In Meckel–Gruber the kidneys are abnormal with multiple cysts. Polydactyly, neural tube defects, oligohydramnios, and occipital encephalocele are also features.
- Once detected, the patient should be referred to a fetal medicine unit for further imaging and counseling. Karyotyping should be offered. Fetal MRI should be performed to better delineate the intracranial anatomy. Associated abnormalities should be excluded.
- Genetic counseling should be offered when appropriate.
- For isolated lesions, the prognosis is largely determined by the size of the encephalocele, the amount of herniated cerebral tissue, the degree of ventriculomegaly, the presence of microcephaly, and the presence of other intracranial abnormalities. Large encephaloceles carry a poor prognosis.

4

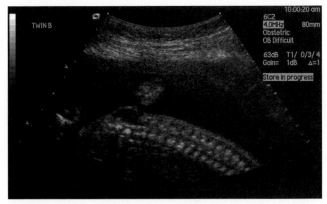

Fig. 4.12. Lubosacral spina bifida.

- Referral to a pediatric neurosurgeon and neurologist for further counseling is essential in cases when continuance of the pregnancy is desired.
- Termination of pregnancy should be offered if the defect is large, if associated malformations are present, aneuploidy, or if a genetic syndrome is detected.
- Caesarean section may be indicated for large lesions to minimize trauma. There is no fetal intervention for this condition.
- Delivery should take place in a tertiary center which has facilities to manage the baby postnatally.
- Postnatally, most encephaloceles will need surgery. In cases of frontal lesions, extensive craniofacial surgery may be required. The long-term outcome is dependent on the degree of herniated brain tissue and the presence of microcephaly. Hydrocephalus develops in a significant proportion of cases and shunting is usually required. The outcome for encephaloceles containing brain tissue is generally poor.

Myelomeningocele
- Most myelomeningoceles occur in the lumbo–sacral region. The lesion contains both neural and meningeal elements that protrude through the defect in the vertebral bones (Figs. 4.12 and 4.13).
- The diagnosis is usually made when a defect is seen in the spine associated with a sac overlying it. In almost 100% of cases the cerebellum is abnormal ("banana" shaped or difficult to visualize) (Fig. 4.14). The skull may also show scalloping of the frontal bones, giving rise to a "lemon" shape appearance. Ventriculomegaly may be present.

CENTRAL NERVOUS SYSTEM ABNORMALITIES

4

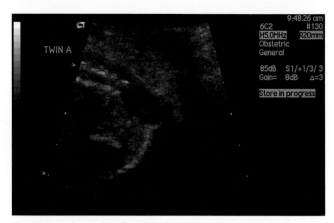

Fig. 4.13. Lumbosacral myelomenigocele.

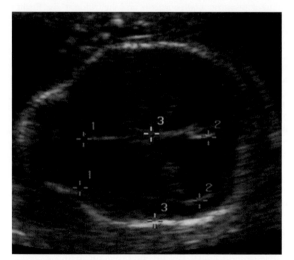

Fig. 4.14. Lemon shaped skull, ventriculomegaly and small cerebellum.

- Differential diagnoses include sacrococcygeal teratoma, lipoma, or other skin masses overlying the spine or caudal regression syndrome.
- Once the diagnosis is suspected, the patient should be referred to a fetal medicine unit for further evaluation. Karyotyping should be

offered. Additional structural anomalies should be excluded. Fetal MRI to assess the spine and brain is useful.

- >80% of fetuses will reach term. Long-term survival following surgery has improved, with >85% of patients surviving at least 5 years.
- Parents must be counseled about some of the long-term health issues which will face survivors and should be given the opportunity of meeting a pediatric neurologist and neurosurgeon to discuss post-natal management and long-term outcome.
- The highest level of the open neural tube determines the degree of muscle dysfunction and paralysis. The lower extremities are completely without muscle function when the lesion is thoracic and there is little useful leg function when the lesion is high lumbar (L1 and L2).
- The number of involved vertebrae, or length of the lesion, or the size of the sac, play no role in determining motor function or have any prognostic significance.
- Kyphosis and severe scoliosis commonly develop when the defect occurs in the thoracic region as the muscular support of the vertebral column itself is deficient.
- The prognosis for lower lesions (L3–L5) for long-term walking and the need for specific orthotic devices are not easy to predict antenatally.
- Patients with sacral lesions have some degree of plantar flexion and will usually be able to ambulate with a very good, although not entirely normal, gait.
- Almost all patients, including those with sacral defects, will have some degree of bowel and bladder dysfunction because the low sacral nerves innervate the distal bowel, anal sphincter, bladder, and internal and external bladder sphincters.
- In addition to being a social problem when the child is not continent, there is also a risk of vesicoureteric reflux and renal damage over time. Surgery is often required.
- Bowel incontinence is a major problem. High-fiber diets, a program of digital stimulation and/or extraction, enemas, or timed evacuation are frequently necessary. Continence surgery may be necessary.
- The Arnold–Chiari type II malformation (brainstem herniation, small posterior fossa, medullary kink, beaked tectum, and a tube-like elongation of the fourth ventricle), is found in almost 100% of patients with a myelocele or myelomeningocele.
- The herniated cerebellum causes an obstruction to the flow of CSF, which may be partial or relatively complete resulting in hydrocephalus. Some degree of hydrocephalus is seen on prenatal ultrasound in 75% of cases. In the majority of patients who have no antenatal ventriculomegaly, hydrocephalus develops soon after the defect is closed. However, approximately 10%–15% of patients will not develop hydrocephalus severe enough to require treatment. Lower lesions are less likely to develop hydrocephalus requiring shunting.

4

CENTRAL NERVOUS SYSTEM ABNORMALITIES

- 85%–90% of children with progressive ventricular enlargement require placement of a ventricular peritoneal shunt. Endoscopic third ventriculostomy is possible but is a controversial approach to management of hydrocephalus in children.
- Shunts may need revision because of proximal or distal obstruction, under- or over-drainage, infection, or mechanical failure. In >60% of cases the median time to the first episode of shunt failure was 303 days. Approximately 32% of patients have two episodes of shunt failure. Infection at the time of placement occurs in approximately 15% of cases. Multiple shunt revisions can threaten intellectual development, but shunt infection is the greatest risk.
- Although pressure on the brainstem is improved with ventricular shunting, some children still suffer from cerebellar and upper cervical nerve dysfunction with problems in oromotor function, swallowing, vocal cord motion, and upper extremity function. Occasional life-threatening central hypoventilation and/or apnea, or vocal cord paralysis and airway obstruction can result.
- The severity of symptoms frequently does not correlate with the degree of hindbrain herniation, making it difficult to predict antenatally which children will be at risk. Children who do not require ventricular shunting have a much better outlook in terms of intelligence. The rate of profound mental retardation (IQ below 20) in those with shunts is approximately 5% and the average IQ is about 80 (low normal range). Profound mental handicap is usually the result of significant medical complications such as shunt infection or severe problems secondary to the Arnold–Chiari II malformation, such as apnea or chronic hypercarbia and/or hypoxia.
- Management of Myelomeningocele Study (MOMS) is an on-going randomized trial designed to investigate the risks and potential benefits of in-utero closure of the spinal defect.
- There is some evidence to suggest that partial hind brain regression may occur following fetal surgery. However, whether this translates into improved long-term respiratory outcome is unclear. There is a significant reduction (45% vs 95%) in the need for shunting in cases treated in utero. This reduction is most marked in fetuses <25 weeks, a lesion below L2 and with ventricles <14 mm. At the present time, there does not appear to be any difference in sensori-motor function of the lower limbs or in bladder/bowel continence in cases compared with controls. Early spinal cord tethering has been noted in babies treated in utero.

THORACIC ABNORMALITIES

Thoracic abnormalities

Fetal lung development

- Pulmonary development requires normal fetal breathing movements, an adequate intra-thoracic space, sufficient amniotic fluid, normal intra-lung fluid volume, and pulmonary blood flow. Maternal health, including nutrition, endocrine factors, smoking, and disease, can also adversely influence lung development.
- There are five stages of lung development:
  1. Embryonic (0–7 weeks in utero)
  2. Pseudoglandular (7–17 weeks in utero)
  3. Canalicular (17–27 weeks in utero)
  4. Saccular (28–36 weeks in utero)
  5. Alveolar (36 weeks in utero–2 years postnatal)

Changes at birth

- Prior to labor, lung fluid secretion falls and the onset of labor stimulates the production of adrenaline by the fetus and thyrotrophin-releasing hormone by the mother, causing fetal pulmonary epithelial cells to begin re-absorption of lung fluid.
- After birth, there is an acceleration of active pulmonary fluid absorption, and most is cleared from the full-term newborn lung within 2 h of commencing spontaneous breathing. This is achieved by the active transport of sodium ions out of the alveolar lumen and into the interstitium. With the introduction of air into the lungs, an air/liquid interface, facilitated by surfactant, forms the alveolar lining.
- After birth, there is a dramatic fall in pulmonary arteriolar resistance and an increase in pulmonary blood flow when the lungs are inflated.
- Once the alveoli are aerated, breathing needs less effort, requiring minimal negative intra-thoracic pressure to maintain a normal tidal volume (Laplace's law).
- Tactile stimulation and the change in temperature that occurs after birth are also potent stimulants for the transition to extrauterine respiration.

Diaphragmatic hernia

- Congenital diaphragmatic hernia (CDH) has an incidence of 1:3000–1:5000 births. The combination of abnormalities associated with CDH, including lung hypoplasia, lung dysmaturity, and pulmonary hypertension can result in high mortality.
- CDH occurs when there is failure of the pleuroperitoneal canal to partition at 9–10 weeks of gestation. This results in herniation of abdominal viscera into the chest causing pulmonary and cardiac compression (Fig. 5.1).

5

THORACIC ABNORMALITIES

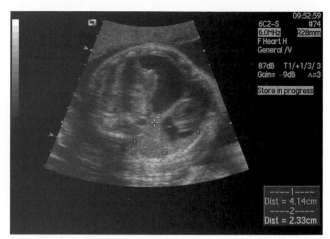

Fig. 5.1. Left diaphragmatic hernia with stomach and small bowel in thorax.

- The degree of pulmonary hypoplasia depends entirely on the length of time and extent the herniated organs have compressed the fetal lungs.
- Associated abnormalities may be present in 30%–60% of cases and can involve any organ system. Aneuploidy is present in 10%–20% of cases and it may also be associated with some genetic syndromes (Fryn's, Beckwith–Wideman syndrome).
- CDH should be suspected if the fetal stomach is not in its usual intra-abdominal position. Liver, mesentery, and bowel and spleen may be present in the chest. Differential diagnoses include congenital cystic adenomatoid malformations, bronchogenic cysts, pulmonary seques-tration, or thoracic teratomas.
- Polyhydramnios and/or hydrops may sometimes be present. Increased liquor is usually due to impaired swallowing and hydrops may occur if there is significant cardiac compression.
- Liver herniation is a poor predictive factor for the development of pulmonary hypoplasia. Attempts have been made to assess the degree of lung hypoplasia using conventional 2D ultrasound, 3D ultra-sound, and fetal MRI. The results are variable, with some studies suggesting better correlation with actual lung volume and therefore outcome using 3D ultrasound and MRI.
- The lung–head ratio (LHR) is commonly used to predict survival in CDH. The LHR is measured at the level of the four chamber view of the heart (area of the lung divided by the head circum-ference). In general, a LHR of <1 is associated with poor survival rates (10%).

5

- LHR increases with gestation and it may be preferable to use the observed to expected normal mean for gestation (O/E) LHR to obtain a gestation-independent prediction of postnatal survival.
- Fetal intervention is possible using fetoscopic tracheal occlusion techniques. The rationale for treatment is the experimental and clinical observations that fetal tracheal occlusion increases lung dry weight, airway branching and promotes pulmonary vascular growth.
- Tracheal occlusion affects lung growth during the canalicular and especially saccular stages, a period critical to lung development as the functional gas exchange units first begin to appear. It amplifies mechanical stretching of lung parenchyma by preventing the normal egress of lung fluid.
- Although there is good theoretical, experimental, and observational basis for tracheal occlusion as a treatment, this has not shown to be the case in a recent randomized controlled trial, which suggested that there was no difference in survival in fetuses treated in utero (73%) compared with babies that received standard neonatal care (77%). There was a higher incidence of premature membrane rupture and preterm delivery in the fetal intervention group.
- Tracheal occlusion may have a role in fetuses with liver herniation and LHR<1. In these cases survival may be improved from 10% to 40%–50% after fetal treatment.
- Management of cases must include detailed assessment of the fetus for additional anomalies. Karyotyping and fetal echocardiography should be performed.
- Fetal MRI or 3D ultrasound should be considered to evaluate lung volume. Parents should be counseled by a pediatric surgeon regarding neonatal management.
- Termination of pregnancy is an option if significant visceral herniation (particularly liver) and early diagnosis.
- Serial scans to assess lung growth and liquor volume is necessary. Development of polyhydramnios suggests some impairment to fetal swallowing and increases risk of preterm labor.
- Aim to deliver at term. Mode of delivery is made on standard obstetric grounds. Essential that delivery takes place in tertiary centre.
- Postdelivery, the baby will need close monitoring to assess degree of pulmonary compromise (hypoplasia and vascular hypertension) before surgery is undertaken.
- In selected cases inhaled nitric oxide or the use of prostacyclin may be of benefit if pulmonary hypertension is problematic.
- Primary closure of the diaphragm is possible if the defect is small, otherwise a synthetic mesh may be required. Postsurgery, total parenteral nutrition may be required for some time before alimentary feeding is established.
- Postmortem essential after perinatal death or termination of pregnancy. Genetic counseling required if Fryn's syndrome (recurrence risk 25%) is diagnosed.

5

Cystic congenital adenomatoid malformation (CCAM)

- CCAMs are characterized by lack of normal alveoli and excessive proliferation and cystic dilatation of terminal respiratory bronchioles. The incidence of CCAM is between 1 in 11 000 and 1 in 35 000 live births and is slightly more common in males.
- CCAMs are usually unilateral (>85%) and usually involves only one lobe of the lung. 60% are left-sided lesions. They are characterized by abnormal airway patterning during pulmonary development and result from abnormal branching of the immature bronchioles.
- Typically, cystic structures arise from an overgrowth of the terminal bronchioles with a reduction in the number of alveoli.
- Five pathological types have been described: Type 0 – acinar dysplasia, Type I – multiple large cysts or a single dominant cyst, Type II – multiple evenly spaced small cysts, Type III – mainly solid mass, Type IV – mainly peripheral cysts. Type II lesions are frequently associated with other structural malformations. There is an increased incidence of cardiac abnormalities (tetralogy of Fallot and truncus arteriosus).
- Arrest in the pseudoglandular phase of lung development (Types I–III) results in a bronchiolar type of epithelium while a later arrest in weeks 22–36 results in an alveolar acinar type (Type IV) of epithelium. CCAMs usually have a direct communication with the tracheobronchial tree.
- Aberrations in the *HOXB-5*, *FGF-7* and *PDGFB* genes have all been implicated in abnormal lung development in CCAM.
- Vascular supply and drainage of CCAMs are derived from the pulmonary system. Some lesions (masses that are histologically and sonographically consistent with CCAMs) have a systemic arterial blood supply similar to that seen in bronchopulmonary sequestration. These are referred to as hybrid lesions.
- Between 45% and 85% of prenatally identified CCAMs will spontaneously regress. However, large macrocystic or solid lesions can cause hydrops, pulmonary hypoplasia, cardiac dysfunction, and perinatal death.
- The majority of fetal CCAMs follow a characteristic growth pattern that is highly dependent on gestational age. There is usually an increase in size between 17 and 26 weeks before slowing down or regressing beyond 30 weeks.
- The diagnosis is usually made on antenatal ultrasound by the detection of enlarged hyperechogenic lungs sometimes containing cysts of varying sizes. Mediastinal shift, cardiac compression, polyhydramnios, and hydrops may also be present.
- The presence of a systemic feeding vessel that distinguishes bronchopulmonary sequestration or a hybrid lesion should be sought. In a hybrid lesion, the feeding vessel tends to arise from the descending aorta.
- Differential diagnoses include any thoracic mass (bronchopulmonary sequestration, bronchogenic or neuroenteric cysts, diaphragmatic hernia, neuroblastoma).

5

THORACIC ABNORMALITIES

- Once a thoracic mass is detected, the patient should be referred to a tertiary fetal medicine unit. The fetus should be examined for any other additional anomalies. Fetal echocardiography should be performed. Karyotyping should be offered.
- An assessment of the size of the CCAM and of the normal lung tissue should be made. Fetal MRI may be helpful. The CCAM volume to head circumference ratio (CVR) allows a gestational age corrected volume ratio to be used prognostically when CCAM lesions are identified. CCAM volume (cm^3) is measured by using the formula for an ellipse (length × height × width × 0.52).
- A CVR is obtained by dividing the CCAM volume (cm^3) by the head circumference (cm) to correct for differences in the fetal gestational age. High-risk lesions tend to have a CVR greater than 1.6.
- Serial scans are essential to monitor the size of the lesion (particularly macrocystic CCAM), the development of cardiac compression, and/ or hydrops.
- Fetal therapy is indicted in cases of macrocystic CCAM complicated by hydrops or significant mediastinal shift and cardiac compression. In general, a single large cyst lends itself best to thoraco-amniotic shunting. Needle aspiration of CCAM is not useful, as fluid within the cysts rapidly reaccumulates.
- The parents should be counseled by a pediatric surgeon about the postnatal management. The mode of delivery is on standard obstetric ground.
- Postnatally the baby will require careful monitoring and a chest X-ray. Surgery may be deferred for up to 24 months.
- Many lesions will regress after birth, although may not completely disappear. Recurrent infections and the risk of malignancy (small) are reasons why surgery is performed. The long-term outcome following surgery is usually excellent.

Bronchopulmonary sequestration

- Bronchopulmonary sequestration (BPS) is used to describe a segment of lung that does not have any identifiable connection with the normal tracheobronchial tree, and which receives its arterial supply from one or more systemic arteries (from the aorta in 80% of cases), rather than from the pulmonary vessels.
- An intralobar sequestration results from early ectopic lung budding prior to pleural development and does not have a separate pleural covering. An extralobar sequestration is a mass of pulmonary paren-chyma with a distinct pleural covering separating it from the adjacent normal tissues.
- The incidence is estimated at 1 per 1000 births with intralobar having an equal male to female ratio and extralobar having a male/ female ratio of four to one.
- Intralobar lesions are more common (75%) and are usually located at the lung bases. 10% have associated anomalies including diaphrag-matic hernia, tracheoesophageal fistula, congenital heart defects,

5

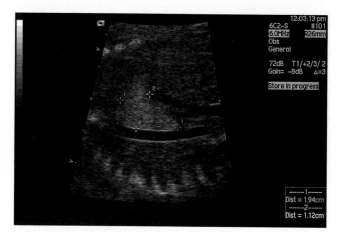

Fig. 5.2. Pulmonary sequestration.

foregut duplication, and aneuploidy. Venous drainage for the intralobar BPS is usually via the pulmonary veins.

- 10% of extralobar lesions are located below the diaphragm. The majority (80%) of extralobar lesions are at the left lung base (Fig. 5.2) and there is an increased incidence (>60%) of associated anomalies.
- Venous drainage is usually via the subdiaphragmatic veins into the systemic circulation. Pleural effusions can be present in 6%–10% of cases.
- The differential diagnoses include CCAM, diaphragmatic hernia, mediastinal hamartoma, neuroblastoma, or bronchogenic cysts.
- If suspected, referral to a tertiary unit should be done. Fetal echocardiography and karyotyping should be performed. Serial scans to assess evolution of the thoracic mass should be performed. Fetal MRI is frequently helpful.
- Intrathoracic lesions can cause mediatsinal shift, cardiac compression, hydrops, and pulmonary hypoplasia. The development of hydrops is a very poor prognostic sign. Intra–abdominal lesions rarely cause antenatal problems.
- Mode of delivery is on standard obstetric grounds. Some neonates may have significant respiratory embarrassment at birth.
- Most cases of extralobar lesions become symptomatic by 6 months of age. Symptoms are rare before the age of 2 years for intralobar BPS. The main complication is recurrent chest infections.
- Resection of intralobar lesions almost always involves a lobectomy. Segmental resection may be possible in some lesions if detected before infection supervenes.

5

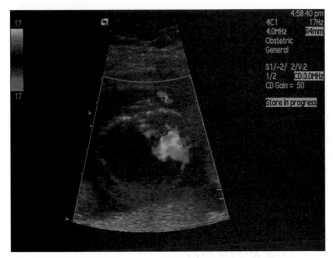

Fig. 5.3. Right pleural effusion with mediastinal shift. See color plate section.

- For extralobar sequestrations, sequestrectomy is often possible. The critical part of the surgical procedure is identification and control of the aberrant vascular supply. The long-term outcome is usually good, although sequelae such as pneumonia, asthma, gastro-esophageal reflux, pectus excavatum, and pyloric stenosis have all been reported.

Pleural effusion

- Fetal pleural effusions have an incidence of between 1 in 10 000–15 000 pregnancies. Effusions may be primary (due to leak of chyle into the pleural cavity) or secondary (seen in hydrops).
- The diagnosis is easily made on antenatal ultrasound (Fig. 5.3). Complications include mediastinal shift, cardiac compression, hydrops, and pulmonary hypoplasia. Affected fetuses are at significant risk for respiratory distress at birth.
- Once detected, the patient should be referred to a fetal medicine unit for further investigations. The presence of other anomalies should be excluded. Fetal echocardiography should be performed. Cardiac abnormalities are present in 5% of cases. Karyotyping should be offered as there is a significant association (10%) with aneuploidy. Maternal serology for infection should be performed.
- Serial scans should be arranged to assess the size of the effusion. The development of hydrops or polyhydramnios is a poor prognostic feature.

THORACIC ABNORMALITIES

5

THORACIC ABNORMALITIES

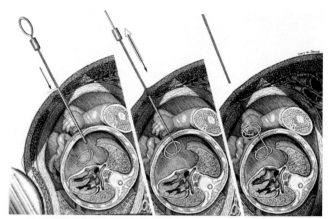

Fig. 5.4. Insertion of a pleuro-amniotic shunt.

- There are several treatment options. First, a period of expectant observation is reasonable if the fetus is not hydropic and the effusion is small or moderate in size.
- Thoracocentesis is simple and can be performed repeatedly. In some cases effusions resolve completely after several aspirations. There is a procedure-related risk with each aspiration and the cumulative risk may be significant if many procedures are required.
- Pleuro-amniotic shunting is another option early in pregnancy. The insertion of a shunt allows drainage of the effusion from the pleural cavity into the amniotic sac (Fig. 5.4). This allows expansion of the lung to occur, improvement in mediastinal shift and cardiac compression, and resolution of the hydrops.
- In the absence of hydrops survival rates are almost 60%. If hydrops is present, survival is only 10%
- Thoracocentesis can also be used just prior to delivery to allow lung expansion, thereby minimizing the need for neonatal resuscitation.
- The pleural fluid should be sent for viral studies and karyotyping.
- The risks associated with pleuro-amniotic shunting include, miscarriage or preterm labor, rupture of membranes, and infection. Additional complications that have been reported include cardiac trauma, blockage of the shunt, internal migration of the shunt requiring thoracotomy for removal after birth and displacement of the shunt. Survival after pleuro-amniotic shunting is approximately 80%.
- In refractory cases, pleurodesis is an option. There have been case reports describing the use of OK-432 (a lyophilized form of an avirulent strain of streptococcal cells with glycolytic and enzymatic properties), which causes the two layers of pleura to adhere to each other. Maternal blood has also been used to achieve the same effect.

5

- If polyhydramnios develops, amnioreduction may be required. In euploid fetuses, if the effusion is isolated, delivery should be considered beyond 32 weeks. At delivery, the shunt must be clamped before the baby takes its first breath, otherwise a pneumothorax may ensue.
- Termination of pregnancy should be offered in cases of aneuploidy, associated major anomalies, progressive hydrops, or non-response to fetal therapy. Most isolated pleural effusions resolve after delivery.

THORACIC ABNORMALITIES

6 ANTERIOR ABDOMINAL WALL DEFECTS

Abdominal wall defects

- Embryologically, four separate folds (cephalic, caudal, and right and left lateral), each of which has a splanchnic and somatic aspect, form the anterior abdominal wall. As this occurs, fetal bowel migrates outside the abdominal cavity through the umbilical ring into the umbilical cord from the 6th to the 11th week of pregnancy.
- The bowel then returns to the abdomen in a stereotypical fashion by 11 weeks, resulting in normal rotation and subsequent fixation.

Omphalocele (exomphalos)

- This is a midline anterior abdominal wall defect of variable size characterized by the absence of abdominal muscles, fascia and skin (Fig. 6.1). It can occur in the upper, mid, or lower abdomen.
- A defect in cranial folding results in a high or epigastric omphalocele classically seen in pentalogy of Cantrell (epigastric omphalocele, anterior diaphragmatic defect, sternal cleft, and pericardial/cardiac defects). Lateral folding defects result in a mid-abdominal omphalocele and caudal defects cause a hypogastric omphalocele seen in bladder or cloacal exstrophy.
- The herniated viscera are covered by a membrane consisting of peritoneum on the inner surface, amnion on the outer surface, and Wharton's jelly between the two layers.
- The umbilical cord inserts into the sac and not into the body wall. Organs commonly in the sac include mesentery, stomach, small and large bowel, and varying amounts of liver, although very large defects can result in extrusion of almost the entire fetal abdominal contents.
- It has an incidence of 1.5–3 per 10 000 births. Most cases are sporadic and are associated with advanced maternal age.
- May occur in isolation or associated with aneuploidy (40%) or as part of a genetic syndrome. Smaller defects are more likely to be associated with chromosome abnormalities.
- Associated abnormalities are common (50%–70%), with cardiac lesions predominating, occurring in 30%–40% of cases. Fetal mortality is strongly associated with the presence of additional malformations.
- Beckwith–Wideman syndrome (omphalocele–macroglossia–gigantism syndrome) occurs in 1 in 13 500 live births. It is characterized by the presence of an omphalocele, macroglossia, organomegaly, and severe neonatal hypoglycemia. It is associated with duplication of chromosome 11p15. Malignant tumors (Wilm's tumor, hepatoblastoma, neuroblastoma) can occur in 10% of cases.
- The diagnosis can be made in the first trimester, although most are detected at mid trimester anomaly scan.

6

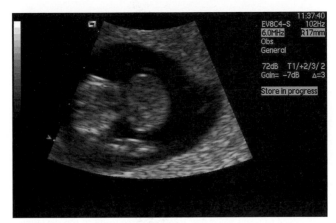

Fig. 6.1. Large omphalocele containing liver and bowel.

ANTERIOR ABDOMINAL WALL DEFECTS

- Maternal serum AFP is usually raised by an average of 4 MoM, although within a wide range. In contrast, gastroschisis is associated with much higher levels (>9 MoM). In general, maternal serum AFP is a poor screening test for abdominal wall defects as the diagnosis is very easily made by ultrasound.
- Once the abnormality has been detected, the patient should be referred to a tertiary center where there are facilities for detailed evaluation of the fetus.
- Offer karyotyping and fetal echocardiography in view of the high association with aneuploidy and cardiac anbormalities.
- Careful assessment of the fetus is necessary to look for additional anomalies. If macroglossia and other organomegaly are detected, Beckwith–Wideman syndrome should be suspected and the cytogenetics laboratory alerted to specifically look for abnormalities in the 11p15 region.
- Multidisciplinary counseling with pediatric surgeons, neonatologists, pediatric cardiologists, and perinatologists is essential. Offer genetic counseling if a genetic syndrome is suspected.
- Offer termination of pregnancy if fetus is aneuploid or if other major malformations are detected.
- Counsel parents about increased incidence of fetal growth restriction, preterm labor, and intrauterine death.
- Delivery should take place in a tertiary centre. Although vaginal delivery is reasonable and does not appear to influence outcome, elective cesarean section may be preferable in order that delivery takes place in a more controlled environment and timing of neonatal surgery can be better planned. Large omphaloceles are probably best delivered by cesarean section because of the possibility of trauma or soft tissue dystocia during a vaginal delivery.

- The risk of recurrence depends on the etiology of the omphalocele. Most isolated cases are sporadic and therefore the risk of recurrence is not increased. Familial cases may have a much higher risk approaching 50% and genetic counseling is essential.
- In both gastroschisis and omphalocele, the aim of surgery is to reduce the herniated viscera into the abdomen and to close the fascia and skin to create a solid abdominal wall with a relatively normal umbilicus. Treatment can, however, vary, depending on the size and type of the defect, the size of the baby, and any associated neonatal problems.
- Most surgeons prefer primary closure whenever possible. However, large defects with significant visceral herniation may require a more gradual or phased approach using silos to achieve a reduction over a period of time before the abdominal wall is finally closed.

Gastroschisis

- Believed to result secondary to an ischemic insult to the developing abdominal wall. There is a full thickness defect that occurs secondary to incomplete closure of the lateral folds during the sixth week of gestation.
- The right paraumbilical area is usually affected. This area is supplied by the right umbilical vein and right omphalomesenteric artery and may be vulnerable if there is premature disruption in these vessels which may predispose to abdominal wall ischemia. An alternative hypothesis that may account for some cases of gastroschisis is that the defect results from an early rupture of a hernia of the umbilical cord.
- The incidence of gastroschisis is between 0.4 and 3 per 10 000 births and appears to be increasing. It has a strong association with young maternal age (<20 years), cigarette smoking, illicit drugs (cocaine), vasoactive over-the-counter drugs (such as pseudoephedrine), and environmental toxins. These associations are all consistent with the vascular disruption/ischemia theory of this abnormality.
- The diagnosis is usually obvious on ultrasound, with free floating bowel or rarely liver evident floating in the amniotic fluid without a covering membrane (Fig. 6.2). Differential diagnosis include, ruptured omphalocele sac or limb–body wall complex. The limb–body wall complex usually has a short umbilical cord and numerous other malformations.
- Associated anomalies occur in 10%–20% of cases and most of these are in the gastrointestinal tract. Approximately 10% of babies have intestinal stenosis or atresia that usually results from vascular interruption to the bowel at the time of gastroschisis development or from later volvulus or compression of the mesenteric vascular pedicle by a narrowing abdominal wall ring. Other rarer anomalies include undescended testes, Meckel's diverticulum, and intestinal duplications.
- Chromosomal abnormalities or genetic syndromes are very rare. There is a slight increase in the incidence of cardiac abnormalities, but this is not as high as seen in omphalocele.

6

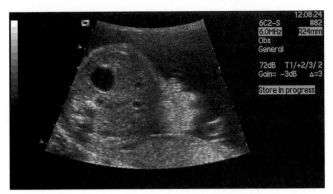

Fig. 6.2. Gastroschisis (note the absence of a covering membrane).

ANTERIOR ABDOMINAL WALL DEFECTS

- There is an increased incidence of preterm labor (30%), fetal growth restriction (70%), oligohydramnios (25%), and fetal death. The cause of fetal growth failure is unclear, but could be partially due to increased protein loss from the exposed viscera.
- The herniated bowel is at risk from volvulus and long segment necrosis and/or more localized atretic and stenotic segments. Bowel that is exposed to amniotic fluid can also develop an inflammatory "peel" or serositis that can cause loops of bowel to adhere to each other making neonatal surgery difficult. This "peel" usually develops after 30 weeks gestation and is difficult to quantify on prenatal ultrasound.
- Increasing bowel dilation, progressive oligohydramnios, or decreased growth velocity may all be indicative of a fetus that is at increased risk of intrauterine death or greater neonatal complications.
- Early referral to a tertiary center with multidisciplinary management is essential.
- Because of the extremely low incidence of aneuploidy, karyotyping is not essential. Fetal echocardiography should be performed due to the increased association with cardiac anomalies.
- Counsel patients about increased incidence of growth restriction, preterm labor and intrauterine death.
- Serial scans to assess fetal growth and liquor volume, degree of bowel dilatation and bowel wall thickness is important.
- No contraindication for vaginal delivery but, as for omphalocele, elective cesarean section may also be an option to facilitate neonatal care.
- Parents need to be aware of surgical management and of some of its potential complications. Overall survival is good (90%–95%), with most deaths occurring in babies who have significant bowel loss, sepsis, or long-term complications of short bowel syndrome.
- There is a 10% risk of hypoperistalsis syndrome, which may require longer hospitalization and hyperalimentation. Gastrointestinal reflux

6

occurs in 10% of cases and there is a 5%–10% risk of obstruction due to adhesions in the longer term. A significant number of cases will also develop inguinal hernias due to increased intra-abdominal pressure postsurgery.

- Counsel parents that the risk of recurrence is small, but exposure to vasoactive substances should be avoided in any subsequent pregnancy.

Body stalk anomaly/limb–body wall complex

- Body stalk anomaly is an extremely rare malformation usually characterized by the presence of a major anterior abdominal wall defect, limb deformities, kyphoscoliosis, an absent or short umbilical cord, and/or craniofacial defects.
- Differential diagnosis includes the amniotic band syndrome, gastroschisis, omphalocele, bladder exstrophy, or the limb–body wall complex.
- Body stalk anomaly may be due to faulty folding in all three axes with persistence of the extra-embryonic celomic cavity. The various malformations associated with body stalk anomaly depend on the degree of aberrant development of each of the four folds.
- Amniotic bands are present in 40% of cases. Some authors believe that early amnion rupture and subsequent partial extrusion of the fetus into the celomic cavity is responsible for the spectrum of abnormalities. There is an increased incidence in monozygotic twins probably due to early embryonic cleavage aberrations.
- Both conditions are sporadic in nature, seen in younger mothers, and usually not associated with aneuploidy.
- If suspected, the patient should be referred to a tertiary center for detailed evaluation of the fetus. The prognosis is dismal with an extremely high incidence of miscarriage, preterm labor and intrauterine death. Neonatal demise is invariable.
- There is no increased risk in subsequent pregnancies.

Bladder exstrophy
- This is a rare defect, with a prevalence of 1 in 30 000 live births.
- It is associated with other anomalies of the anterior abdominal wall, perineum, genitalia, and bony pelvis. The pubic rami are everted with some degree of diastasis and there is outward rotation and splaying of the innominate bones.
- The diagnosis is suspected when the normal intrapelvic bladder is not visualized, a low anterior abdominal wall mass is present, genital abnormalities (short penis), low umbilical cord insertion, and splaying of the pelvic bones is present.
- Differential diagnoses includes cloacal exstrophy, omphalocele, and gastroschisis.
- Vesico-ureteric reflux is present in 90% of cases. Surviving patients may have life-long problems of chronic urinary incontinence, sexual

dysfunction, increased risk of adenocarcinoma of the bladder, and renal failure.

- Termination of pregnancy should be discussed with parents if the diagnosis is made early. This may still be an option later in gestation, but the parents should be fully counseled by a pediatric urologist.
- The aims of reconstructive surgery in patients with bladder exstrophy are to maintain kidney function, achieve urinary continence, and to create or preserve functionally normal external genitalia.
- Complications associated with surgery might take many years to become evident. Sexual function, fertility, and self-esteem are additional long-term issues in treated patients. Although favorable results in terms of renal function and cosmetic appearance have been achieved with staged reconstruction, persistent urinary incontinence is a common complication.
- Primary neonatal repair is another option and may have a beneficial impact on renal function and continence, although 50% of patients will need further surgery to deal with reflux and epispadias revisison.
- In patients with untreated bladder extrophy, adenosarcoma of the bladder is common.

Cloacal exstrophy

- Cloacal exstrophy is the rarest and most extreme form of the exstrophy anomalies and has an incidence of 1 in 200 000–1 in 400 000 births.
- Failure of the caudal fold to close results in cloacal exstrophy. Classically, it consists of an exstrophic central bowel field flanked by two hemi-bladders. In addition, an infraumbilical omphalocoele is present in 90% of cases. Frequently, anal atresia, hypoplasia of the colon, and genital anomalies (absent penis/clitoris or scrotum, epispadias, hemiscrotum), as well as neural tube defects are present in 50% of cases.
- The terminal ileum often prolapses through a proximal orifice in the ileocaecal region, producing an elephant trunk deformity. The distal orifice leads to a short, blind-ending segment of colon.
- Additional structural anomalies in other organ systems are present in 85% of cases. Urinary tract and vertebral anomalies are particularly common.
- The term OEIS complex (omphalocele, exstrophy of bladder, imperforate anus, spinal defects) is also used to describe the features associated with exstrophy of the cloaca.
- On ultrasound, cloacal exstrophy should be suspected when a lower anterior abdominal wall defect is present, together with absence of a normal bladder. Splaying of the pubic rami and neural tube defects are also frequently present and help support the diagnosis. The elephant trunk deformity caused by prolapse of the ileum may also be seen.
- Differential diagnoses include bladder exstrophy, isolated infraumbilical omphalocele, gastroschisis, amniotic band syndrome, and the limb–body wall complex. In amniotic band syndrome and limb–body wall

complex, the infraumbilical omphalocele and neural tube defect is usually absent.

- There is an increased incidence of miscarriage, preterm labor, and intrauterine death. Polyhydramnios is not infrequent.
- If the diagnosis is made antenatally, the parents must be offered the option of termination of pregnancy. Fetal karyotype is usually normal. If continuance of the pregnancy is desired, the patient should be referred to a tertiary center with facilities for both fetal medicine expertise as well as neonatal surgical experience to deal with this challenging abnormality.
- This condition often is compatible with extra-uterine life, but requires multiple complex surgeries for survival. The management of children with cloacal exstrophy has improved remarkably, and most series suggest that approximately 90% of affected babies are now surviving into childhood and beyond. Complex reconstruction should only be performed in tertiary centers with experience in dealing with this type of major multi-system abnormality.
- Bladder reconstruction, gender reassignment, and vaginal recon-struction, pelvic and spinal surgery as well as major gastrointestinal surgery are required. Long-term problems include urinary (low bladder compliance and capacity, reflux, calculi formation), short bowel syndrome, psychological adjustment, impaired sexual function, fertility, and quality of life issues.

Urorectal septum malformation sequence (URSMS)
- This is characterized by absent perineal and anal openings, ambiguous or absent external genitalia, and urogenital anomalies. It is also associ-ated with cardiac, gastrointestinal, vertebral, and limb abnormalities.
- Pulmonary hypoplasia due to oligohydramnios and renal abnormalities are common. Unlike bladder and cloacal exstrophy, the full URSMS is not compatible with postnatal life.
- Theories as to the etiology of URSMS include abnormalities of fusion of the urorectal septum membrane with the cloacal membrane and deficiency of caudal mesoderm.

GASTROINTESTINAL AND BILIARY TRACT ABNORMALITIES

- Mammalian gastrointestinal epithelium is derived from embryonic endoderm, whereas the muscular, hematopoietic and connective tissue components are derived from mesoderm. The tubular structure of the intestine is created by folding of the endodermal layer, and is accompanied by changes in gene expression along the anterior–posterior axis resulting in ventral–dorsal patterning and formation of the foregut (duodenum, liver and pancreas), midgut, and hindgut.
- Rapid cellular proliferation of the endoderm and mesenchyme results in elongation of the bowel. This is accompanied by a complex series of rotational events that result in the proper positioning of the gut within the abdominal cavity.
- Differentiation of the endoderm into the mature epithelium occurs in concert with this process, resulting in the mature intestinal epithelium exhibiting regional differences in morphology and function from duodenum to ileum.
- The total small bowel length is 250 cm in a term neonate and 160–240 cm in a preterm neonate.
- Fetal or neonatal intestinal obstruction often manifests itself with a number of signs, including maternal polyhydramnios, bilious vomiting, abdominal distension, and failure to pass meconium in the first 24 h of life.

Duodenal atresia

- At 5 weeks of embryonic life, the lumen of the duodenum is obliterated by proliferating epithelium. Luminal patency is usually restored by the 11th week and any aberration in canalisation may lead to stenosis or atresia.
- Duodenal atresia has an incidence of 1 in 5000–10 000 live births. The diagnosis is suspected on ultrasound when polyhydramnios and a double bubble appearance (due to a dilated stomach and proximal duodenum) (Fig. 7.1) are present. Although occasionally seen earlier in gestation, the diagnosis is usually only made after 24 weeks.
- Approximately 50% of cases of duodenal atresia have associated anomalies. 30% are associated with Down syndrome and other anomalies are usually related to the VACTERL group (Vertebral, Anorectal, Cardiac, TracheoEsophageal, Renal and Limb).
- Differential diagnoses for a double bubble appearance include duodenal obstruction from an annular pancreas, malrotation or volvulus of the midgut, gastric or duodenal duplications. Often, the diagnosis is only apparent during neonatal surgery.
- Postnatal symptoms depend on the type and degree of obstruction with most cases presenting with bilious vomiting soon after birth. In about 10% of cases, the obstruction is pre-ampullary and the

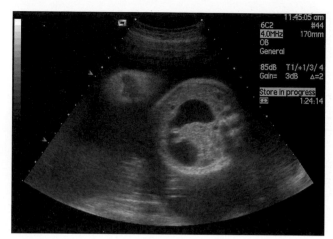

Fig. 7.1. Duodenal atresia with double bubble appearance.

vomiting is non-bilious. An abdominal X-ray with a double bubble appearance and no distal bowel gas is usually diagnostic of duodenal atresia.

- After birth, a nasogastric tube should be placed to prevent aspiration of gastric contents and gastric perforation. Once the neonate has been resuscitated, operative correction is performed with the aim of treatment being to restore continuity of the proximal bowel. The procedure of choice is a duodenoduodenostomy or occasionally a duodenojejunostomy. Survival rates following surgery is now in excess of 90%, and mortality in most cases is due to associated anomalies.
- Long-term problems include the blind loop syndrome, duodenal–gastric or gastroesophalgeal reflux, cholelithiasis, and cholecystitis.
- Most euploid cases are sporadic with minimal recurrence risk.
- If the diagnosis is suspected on antenatal ultrasound, karyotyping must be offered because of the high risk of Down syndrome. Careful survey of the fetus for other structural anomalies is also required. If aneuploidy is confirmed, termination of pregnancy is an option.
- Because of the significant risk of polyhydramnios (50%) frequent scans are required and amnioreduction offered if the amniotic fluid index is ≥40 cm or if the patient is symptomatic. Preterm labor occurs in approximately 40% of cases.
- Delivery should take place in a tertiary center with neonatal and pediatric surgical facilities.

Midgut malrotation and volvulus
- The midgut is the segment of bowel that herniates into the extra-embryonic celomic cavity in the early first trimester. It rotates 90° as

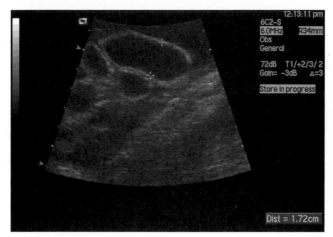

Fig. 7.2. Severe bowel dilatation.

it herniates into the yolk sac and another 270° as it re-enters the embryonic celomic cavity.

- The incidence of malrotation is about 1 in 6000 live births and is a neonatal surgical emergency. 50% of cases present in the neonatal period.
- A failure of rotation at any point can result in the cacum not properly located in the right lower quadrant. The mesentery, which is fixed at only one point behind the superior mesenteric axis, may twist on itself, leading to a midgut volvulus. Because the mesentery contains the superior mesenteric vessels which supply and drain the small intestine, bowel necrosis may occur very quickly. Delay in surgery can result in significant morbidity with loss of much of the midgut due to strangulation and necrosis.
- Significant bowel dilatation on antenatal ultrasound should be carefully monitored and the baby reviewed by a pediatric surgeon soon after birth.

Intestinal atresias
- Approximately 30% of neonates presenting with intestinal obstruction have atresia or stenosis (Fig. 7.2). The exact etiology is unclear, but is postulated to be as a result of a localized intrauterine vascular accident with ischemic necrosis of the sterile bowel and subsequent resorption of the affected segment.
- Common sites include the distal ileum (35%), proximal jejunum (30%), distal jejunum (20%), and proximal ileum (15%). In about 10% of cases multiple atretic segments are present.

- The diagnosis of obstruction secondary to atresia is usually made after 25 weeks as intestinal dilatation is slow and progressive. There is also a lower incidence of associated anomalies.
- Intestinal atresia is associated with meconium ileus (cystic fibrosis) in 20% of cases, and up to 20% of gastroschisis and omphaloceles have associated bowel atresia.
- High obstruction may cause polyhydramnios. The presence of intra-peritoneal calcifications is indicative of meconium peritonitis and suggests an intrauterine bowel perforation.
- Delivery should take place in a tertiary center with neonatal and pediatric surgical facilities.
- Contrast enemas are usually required to confirm the diagnosis of atresia. Delay in the diagnosis may result in impairment of viability (50%), frank necrosis and perforation (10%–20%), fluid and electro-lyte abnormalities and an increased incidence of sepsis.
- Depending on the findings, resection of the proximal dilated bowel with primary anastomosis is commonly performed. An enter-ostomy is created if there is bowel perforation or if there are concerns about gut viability. Survival rates following surgery are around 85%–90%.
- Long-term complications include hypoperistalsis and long-term requirement for parenteral nutrition and short bowel syndrome.

Meconium ileus/peritonitis
- Meconium ileus is impaction of abnormally thick and sticky meco-nium in the distal ileum. Meconium peritonitis occurs when there is in-utero perforation of bowel resulting in a sterile chemical peritonitis.
- Ultrasound features of meconium peritonitis include intra-abdominal calcifications, hyperechogenic bowel (Fig. 7.3), ascites, and bowel dilatation. Polyhydramnios may also be present.
- Differential diagnoses include hepatic calcifications, congenital infections (cytomegalovirus or toxoplasma) or fetal tumors (neuroblastoma, hepatoblastoma, and teratoma).
- The presence of significant bowel dilatation, ascites, meconium pseudocysts, or ascites usually suggests that neonatal surgery will be required.
- Serial ultrasound scans should be performed to assess progression of bowel dilatation, development of ascites or intra-abdominal cysts, and polyhydramnios, which might indicate complicated meconium peritonitis with a 50% chance of requiring neonatal surgery. If these are present, consideration should be given to delivering the baby in a tertiary center with neonatal surgical facilities.
- Parental cystic fibrosis carrier testing and/or invasive fetal testing should be offered. If cystic fibrosis is diagnosed, appropriate genetic counseling should be offered and termination of pregnancy discussed if the diagnosis is made early in pregnancy.
- Long-term outcome depends on the underling cause for the meconium peritonitis. In simple isolated meconium peritonitis the prognosis is

7

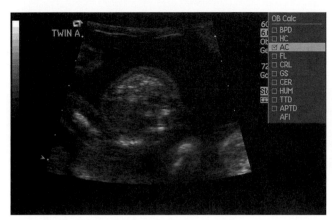

Fig. 7.3. Hyperechogenic bowel.

usually excellent. In infants with cystic fibrosis the long-term outlook is guarded because of other extra-abdominal complications that can develop.

Colonic abnormalities
- Obstruction of the colon in the newborn may be either anatomical or functional. Colonic atresia is rare and accounts for <10% of all cases of intestinal atresias. Prenatal diagnosis is difficult, but should be considered when the large bowel is significantly dilated. Polyhydramnios is uncommon and should raise suspicions about a more proximal obstruction. If perforation occurs, meconium peritonitis and ascites can result.
- The differential diagnoses include anorectal atresia and Hirschprung's disease.
- Hirschsprung's disease occurs in 1:5000 live births and is characterized by an absence of enteric neurons in terminal regions of the gut, leading to tonic contraction of the affected segment, intestinal obstruction and massive distension of the proximal bowel (megacolon). The diagnosis is almost always made in the neonatal period, although antenatal diagnosis has occasionally been described.
- It may be either familial or sporadic, and is classified into two types, depending on the extent of aganglionosis. Short-segment Hirschsprung's occurs most commonly and affects the rectum and a short portion of the colon, whereas long-segment disease affects longer tracts of the colon, and in rare cases presents as total colonic or total intestinal aganglionosis.
- Ten genes and five Hirschsprung's disease susceptibility loci have been identified in humans. The majority of cases are sporadic.

The ratio of male to female patients is 4:1. Although in most cases (70%) it is an isolated trait, it can also occur as part of a number of genetic syndromes. It is also associated with chromosomal abnormalities such as Down syndrome, which accounts for up to 10% of cases.

- Large bowel obstruction is rarely associated with aneuploidy and karyotyping is therefore not indicated. It is also usually not associated with prematurity. Delivery should take place in a center with neonatal surgical facilities.

Choledochal cyst

- Choledochal cysts are rare, congenital cystic dilatations of the biliary tree. They can lead to cholangitis, calculi formation, portal hypertension, and malignancy of the biliary tract. Choledochal cysts have a predilection for females and occur more commonly in patients of Asian descent. Most cases are sporadic.
- Five variants have been described. Type I, is the most common, and is essentially a dilatation of the common bile duct. This is further subdivided into Type IA (marked dilatation of part or all of the extrahepatic bile duct with the gallbladder/cystic duct arising from the cyst), Type IB (focal dilatation of the distal common bile duct) and Type IC (fusiform dilatation of the common bile duct and involves the common hepatic duct). Type II anomaly is a diverticulum of the common bile duct and type III represents a choledochocele, which is found in the intraduodenal portion of the common bile duct. Type IV also includes Type IVA (with both intrahepatic and extrahepatic biliary dilatation) and Type IVB (extrahepatic multisegmental biliary dilatation). Type V or Caroli's disease involves dilatation of the intrahepatic bile ducts.
- The typical antenatal ultrasound finding is a simple cystic structure in the right upper fetal abdomen. Differential diagnoses include gallbladder duplication, mesenteric or duplications cysts, duodenal atresia, hepatic or renal cysts, and dilated loops of bowel.
- The diagnosis of a fetal choledochal cyst should not influence timing or mode of delivery. Patients should be given the opportunity of antenatal surgical counseling and delivery, ideally, should take place in a center with neonatal surgical facilities.
- Cyst excision is recommended as unresected choledochal cysts are associated with an increased risk of subsequent biliary malignancy. Most tumors are cholangiocarcinomas, although squamous cell carcinomas and anaplastic carcinomas can also occur. The risk of carcinoma in children under 10 years old is <1%, but can rise to almost 14% in adults.

GENITOURINARY TRACT ABNORMALITIES

- Congenital anomalies of the kidney and urinary tract account for one-third of all anomalies detected by routine fetal ultrasonography.
- The human kidney (metanephros) develops from the Wolffian duct and the metanephric mesenchyme, which are both derived from the intermediate mesoderm. An outgrowth from the Wolffian duct, called the ureteric bud, invades the metanephric mesenchyme and induces the mesenchymal cells that surround it to condense to form a cap of closely associated cells.
- Mesenchymal aggregation and ureteric bud induction and differentiation depend on mutual interactions mediated by growth factors and matrix molecules, with transcription factors controlling expression of the necessary genes.
- The condensed mesenchymal cells undergo a mesenchyme-to-epithelial transition to form an epithelial tubule. These tubules develop into nephrons, the excretory units of the kidney, by means of several stages of development. The branches of the ureteric bud eventually form the collecting-duct system, which collects urine into the renal pelvis and urinary bladder.
- During ureteric-bud branching, tubule induction is repeated to generate approximately 500 000–1 000 000 nephrons in the human kidney.
- In humans, fetal glomeruli develop by 8–9 weeks, tubular function commences after the 14th week and nephrogenesis is largely complete by birth. After 20 weeks, the kidneys provide over 90% of the amniotic fluid.
- Any bilateral renal malformation can be associated with oligo/anhydramnios, lung hypoplasia, joint contractures and facial abnormalities collectively termed the *Potter sequence*.
- A range of urinary tract abnormalities can occur (Table 8.1), many due to mutations in transcription factor and growth factor genes (Table 8.2).
- Most cases of fetal renal abnormalities present with either enlarged hyperechogenic kidneys (+/− cysts) or hydronephrosis.

Hydronephrosis
- The purpose of the ultrasound scan is to ascertain if the hydronephrosis is isolated or associated with other urological or structural abnormalities. It is important to assess severity and if it is unilateral or bilateral.
- If possible, the level of obstruction should be assessed (i.e. pelvi-ureteric, vesico–ureteric, or lower urinary tract obstruction (LUTO)). Ureteric dilatation and/or bladder enlargement (including bladder wall thickness) should be assessed. Vesico-ureteric reflux can also present with either unilateral or bilateral hydronephrosis, especially in male fetuses.

8

GENITOURINARY TRACT ABNORMALITIES

Table 8.1 *Classification of renal tract malformations*

Malformation	Characteristic(s)
Upper renal tract	
Agenesis	Kidney is absent
Dysplasia	Kidney contains undifferentiated and metaplastic tissues and may be very small (aplasia) and may contain cysts (cystic dysplasia) that may grossly distend the organ (multicystic dysplasia)
Hypoplasia	Kidney contains formed nephrons but significantly fewer than normal; when nephrons are large the condition is called *oligomeganephronia*
Duplex kidney	Kidney is separated into an upper part, which is often dysplastic and attached to an obstructed ureter, and a lower part attached to a ureter with vesico-ureteric reflux
Horseshoe kidney	Both kidneys are fused and may be partly dysplastic
Lower renal tract	
Agenesis	Ureter and bladder trigone is absent; kidney is also absent
Hydronephrosis	Renal pelvis is enlarged and the kidney parenchyma may be hypoplastic or dysplastic; attached ureter may be refluxing or obstructed
Duplication	Partial or complete double ureter may occur with a duplex kidney; insertion into the bladder may be obstructed by a ureterocele
Vesico-ureteric reflux	Urine flows retrogradely from the bladder into the ureter, pelvis, and medullary collecting ducts of the kidney
Posterior urethral valves	Outflow to the urinary bladder is anatomically obstructed; bladder is malformed and kidneys affected by cystic dysplasia

The following birth incidences have been quoted; duplex ureter, 1/120; vesico-ureteric reflux, 1/50–100; horseshoe kidney, 1/200; unilateral renal agenesis, 1/500–1/1000; unilateral multicystic kidney, 1/5000; bilateral agenesis/dysplasia, 1/5000–1/10 000; posterior urethral valves, 1/8000.

Source: Woolf and Winyard 2002, *Paediatric and Developmental Pathology*.

- Severity of the renal pelvic dilatation is assessed by measuring the renal pelvis in antero–posterior plane (>6 mm after 20 weeks is abnormal). Renal pelvic dilatation (RPD) >10 mm represents moderate hydronephrosis and >15 mm is considered severe (Fig. 8.1).
- Calyceal extension, if present, should be documented and cortical thickness measured. Echogenicity of the kidneys and the presence of renal cysts should also be assessed.

Table 8.2 *Mouse mutants and renal tract development*

Gene	Characteristics
Transcription factors	
BF2	Small, fused, and undifferentiated kidneys
EYA1[a]	Absent kidneys
EMX2	Absent kidneys
FOXc1/FOXc2[b]	Urinary tract duplications
HOXa11/HOXd11[b]	Small or absent kidneys
LIM1	Absent kidneys
LMX1B[a]	Malformed glomeruli
N-MYC	Poorly developed mesonephric kidneys
PAX2[a,c]	Small or absent kidneys
WT1[a]	Absent kidneys
Growth factors and receptors	
AT2	A range of kidney and lower urinary tract malformations
EGF receptor	Cystic collecting ducts
BMP4	Malformed kidneys and ureters
BMP7	Undifferentiated kidneys
GDNF[c] and its receptor RET[a]	Small or absent kidneys
PDGF B	Absent mesangial cells
WNT4	Undifferentiated kidneys
Adhesion molecules and receptors	
$\alpha 3$ integrin	Decreased collecting duct branching
$\alpha 8$ integrin	Impaired ureteric bud branching and nephron formation
glypican 3	Deregulated proliferation and apoptosis and renal dysplasia
s-laminin/laminin $\beta 2$	Nephrotic syndrome
Miscellaneous molecules	
BCL2	Small kidneys
COX2	Small kidneys
Formin	Absent kidneys
Neuronal nitric oxide synthase	Bladder outflow obstruction
RAR$\alpha\gamma/\alpha\beta 2$[b]	Small or absent kidneys

Unless otherwise stated, malformations only occur in homozygous null mutants.
[a]Mutations of these genes have also been implicated in malformations of the human renal tract.
[b]Null mutation of two homologous genes is required to cause malformation.
[c]Heterozygous mutations also produce kidney or lower urinary tract malformation.

Source: Woolf and Winyard 2002, *Paediatric & Developmental Pathology*.

8

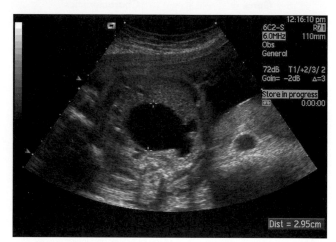

Fig. 8.1. Severe hydronephrosis.

- In isolated cases (either unilateral or bilateral) the risk of aneuploidy is only marginally increased (RR 1.9 for trisomy 21). Karyotyping should be offered in those with an increased a priori risk or if there are additional soft markers/structural anomalies.
- Parents should be counseled that one-third of cases resolve antenatally, especially with mild RPD. A marginally elevated renal pelvic measurement may well be a variant of normal (6–7 mm may be considered a gray zone comprising both mild RPD, and normal babies).
- The overall risk of any pathology (utero-pelvic junction obstruction, vesicoureteric reflux, posterior urethral valves, ureteral obstruction, etc.) is approximately 12% in mild cases, 45% in moderate RPD dilatation, and almost 88% in severe cases.
- A definitive diagnosis can only be made definitively after birth after further investigations. Babies with persistent RPD will require prophylactic antibiotics to prevent urinary tract infection. Most infants will not need surgery (only 20% overall will need pyeloplasty). Surgery is more likely in severe cases.
- Delivery is on standard obstetric grounds and there is usually no need for early delivery.

Renal agenesis
- Unilateral renal agenesis has an incidence of 1 in 500–1000 births compared with bilateral renal agenesis (BRA) which occurs in 1 in 5000–10 000 births. BRA is not compatible with extra-uterine life. It occurs more commonly in males and there is also an increased incidence in twins.

8

- Poorly controlled maternal diabetes or ingestion of reno-toxic drugs are other etiologic factors.
- The diagnosis is usually made at the mid trimester fetal anomaly scan. Although earlier diagnosis is sometimes possible, it is often difficult in the first trimester as the amniotic fluid volume is not significantly reduced at that stage.
- Anhydramnios is usually present by mid trimester in BRA. The liquor volume is usually normal in unilateral agenesis and the normal kidney can be larger due to compensatory hypertrophy.
- Progressive early oligohydramnios or anhydramnios should prompt careful evaluation of the fetal kidneys if membrane rupture has been excluded. Because oligohydramnios can limit visualization of the fetus, color Doppler mapping of the renal arteries can sometimes help in making the diagnosis. These vessels are absent in fetuses with BRA. Occasionally, one of the kidneys may be in an ectopic position.
- There is an increased incidence of additional anomalies, particularly in the genital (blind vagina, uterine malformations, seminal vesicle cysts), cardiovascular, and gastrointestinal systems in up to 44% of fetuses with renal agenesis.
- Contralateral renal abnormalities are common in fetuses with unilateral agenesis. These include multicystic dysplasia, renal hypoplasia, horseshoe kidney, and hydronephrosis.
- Long-term problems in children with isolated unilateral renal agenesis include vesicoureteric reflux, hypertension and proteinuria, although a precise estimate of risk is difficult.
- Renal agenesis (either unilateral or bilateral) can occur in association with genetic syndromes (Fraser, Kallman, branchio-oto-renal, Rokitansky–Kuster–Hauser). A dominant inheritance with incomplete penetrance is postulated in some cases.
- Differential diagnoses include sirenomelia and caudal regression syndrome, which is usually associated with bilateral renal agenesis. Other causes (placental insufficiency, ruptured membranes) for the oligo/anhydramnios must be excluded.
- Amnioinfusion can be performed to improve visualization to confirm the diagnosis of BRA. It, however, has no role in trying to prevent pulmonary hypoplasia and parents should be offered the option of termination of pregnancy.
- A third of fetuses with BRA are still born. Caesarean section is not indicated and babies that are born alive rapidly die from pulmonary hypoplasia and renal failure.
- If the diagnosis of BRA is made antenatally, the parents must be counseled about the dismal outcome and offered termination of pregnancy. Karyotyping and postmortem are essential to help diagnose aneuploidy or a specific syndrome.
- Ultrasound of parental kidneys should be performed.
- Genetic counseling should be offered. The risk of recurrence is low in unilateral renal agenesis 2%–4% but can be as high as 6%–10% in bilateral cases.

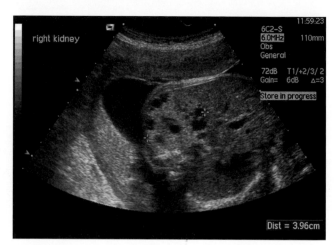

Fig. 8.2. Multicystic dysplastic kidney.

Multicystic dysplastic kidney (MCDK)

• Unilateral MCDK has an incidence of 1 in 3000–5000 live births compared to 1 in 10 000 for bilateral dysplasia. It is one of the commonest causes of an abdominal mass in the neonatal period.

• The abnormal kidneys contain undifferentiated cells and metaplastic elements such as cartilage. Aberrant expression of important nephrogenic transcription factors such as PAX2 and of the pro-apoptotic molecule BCL2, results in dysregulation of cell growth and proliferation in both the epithelial and mesenchymal lineages. The expression of many cytokines and growth factors (hepatocyte growth factor (HGF), Insulin like growth factor (IGF), tumor necrosis factor (TNF) and transforming growth factor (TGF-1)) is also abnormal in dysplastic kidneys.

• On ultrasound, large, hyperechogenic kidneys containing multiple cysts of varying sizes are evident (Fig. 8.2). The cysts are distributed randomly and do not connect. Some kidneys can be massive, distending the entire fetal abdomen. Smaller dysplastic kidneys are more difficult to detect especially in the presence of oligohydramnios. Lower urinary tract obstructive features should be specifically looked for.

• Contra-lateral renal abnormalities can occur in 30%–50% of cases. The prognosis for the fetus depends on whether there is unilateral or bilateral dysplasia. Bilateral MCDK is associated with a similar grim prognosis as BRA, with fetuses dying from pulmonary hypoplasia after birth.

• There is a small risk of long-term hypertension and malignant transformation in the dysplastic kidney.

• MCDK can be associated with aneuploidy (trisomy 13) or various genetic syndromes (Meckel–Gruber, Roberts, Brachial-oto-renal,

8

etc.), which can have either an autosomal dominant or recessive inheritance pattern.

- No specific fetal intervention is required in cases of isolated unilateral MCDK. Serial ultrasound scans to monitor size of the abnormal kidney and liquor volume should be performed. Occasionally, gradual resorption (autonephrectomy) of the abnormal kidney can occur. Karyotyping should be offered to exclude aneuploidy. The mode of delivery is based on standard obstetric grounds. The prognosis is usually good.
- Termination of pregnancy should be offered in cases of bilateral MCDK.
- Fetal postmortem and genetic counseling are important. The risk of recurrence in isolated MCDK is approximately 2%–3%, but may be higher if associated with a genetic syndrome.
- The neonate should receive prophylactic antibiotics and investigated further (micturating cystoureterogram (MCUG), ultrasound, renal function tests, dimercaptosuccinic acid (DMSA) or mercapto acetyl triglycine (MAG-3) scans, etc.).

Lower urinary tract obstruction (LUTO)
- In male fetuses posterior urethral valves (PUV) is the most common cause (90%) of bladder outlet obstruction. In female fetuses urethral atresia accounts for the majority of cases. Oligohydramnios and a large, thick-walled bladder with a keyhole sign (Fig. 8.3) and bilateral hydroureters and hydronephrosis are usually evident on ultrasound.
- PUV consist of a thin membrane of tissue that obstructs the proximal urethra preventing normal egress of urine into the amniotic cavity. It has an incidence of 1 in 8000–25 000 live births.
- Other causes of LUTO are prune belly syndrome and urethral atresia. The prognosis is worse (95% mortality) in those diagnosed antenatally when mid trimester oligohydramnios is present.
- Features that suggest poor prognosis include dilatation of the upper tract, increased bladder wall thickness, oligohydramnios, and evidence of renal dysplasia (echogenic renal cortex and cystic renal change), especially before 24 weeks.
- Obstruction can be complete or partial and the amount of liquor volume usually gives some idea as to the severity of the obstruction. In complete obstruction anhydramnios rapidly develops. In addition, renal dysplasia can occur from an early gestation if the obstruction is severe.
- Dysplastic kidneys associated with obstruction contain undifferentiated and metaplastic tissues such as smooth muscle and cartilage. Some investigators postulate that dysplasia occurs because of increased urinary back pressure on the kidneys causing up-regulation of the transcription factor PAX2 in epithelial tissues and transforming growth factor-1 in mesenchymal tissue resulting in increased stroma and epithelial cyst formation.
- Differential diagnosis of PUV includes urethral atresia, megacystis–microcolon–hypoperistalsis syndrome, obstruction due to a ureterocele

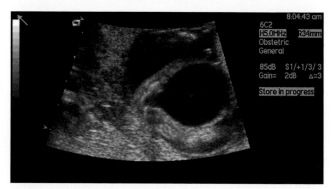

Fig. 8.3. Keyhole sign in obstructed bladder.

or prune-belly syndrome. The megacystis–microcolon–hypoperistalsis syndrome is an autosomal recessive condition and is associated with small bowel dilatation, microcolon, and polyhydramnios. 80% of affected fetuses are female.

- Detailed evaluation of the fetus is important to look for additional anomalies. The appearances of the fetal kidneys may give an idea as to the degree of renal dysplasia and therefore prognosis. Karyotyping is important as aneuploidy is present in up to 10% of cases.
- Termination of pregnancy is an option, particularly if there is severe oligo/anhydramnios, the diagnosis is made early in pregnancy or if there is evidence of renal dysplasia on ultrasound.
- Fetal therapy is possible, although there are no randomized trials as to any particular option's efficacy.
- Treatment can include serial vesicocentesis, percutaneous vesico-amniotic shunting or cystoscopy (experimental).
- The rationale for vesico-amniotic shunting is to decompress the urinary tract and therefore relieve the back pressure on the fetal kidneys and to hopefully prevent the development of renal dysplasia. Shunting also allows restoration of flow of fetal urine into the amniotic cavity and thus prevents pulmonary hypoplasia.
- Fetal urine analysis assists the prognostication of urinary obstruction and therefore the success of fetal therapy. Good prognostic features in fetuses with obstructive uropathies, include urinary sodium <100 Meq/l, chloride <90 Meq/l, osmolality <200 mosml/l and β_2-microglobulin <6 mg/l. These values, however, should be gestationally referenced to be accurate. Urinary sodium and calcium levels are significantly higher in fetuses with renal dysplasia.
- Analysis of serial bladder aspirations may be more representative of renal function than the analysis of a single urine sample from an obstructed fetal bladder. Sequential urine sampling and analysis of urinary electrolytes improve the sensitivity of predicting renal

8

function. Serial sampling is only necessary if the first sample predicts poor outcome.

- A review of five large series involving 169 successfully placed shunts showed that the overall perinatal survival after intervention was only 47%. Shunt-related complications occurred in 45% of cases and included shunt blockage and/or migration, preterm labor, urinary ascites, chorioamnionitis, iatrogenic gastroschisis, and limb contractures.

- Procedure related loss occurs after up to 5% of shunting procedures. Shunting is technically not feasible <17 weeks – before this, serial decompression by urine aspiration may be considered.

- There is rarely any indication to deliver preterm. If there has been a period of prolonged oligohydramnios, pulmonary hypoplasia may preclude neonatal survival. Neonatal investigations include urological consultation, renal ultrasound, MCUG and, on occasion, radionuclide scans.

- The risk of requiring dialysis and subsequent renal failure is approximately 30%–50% in several series. Additional long-term problems include reflux, recurrent infections, bladder compliance, and voiding issues and sexual dysfunction.

- Fetal cystoscopy, which can be both diagnostic and therapeutic, is another potential management option in LUTO. It allows exploration of the bladder and the proximal part of the urethra under endoscopic vision to make the diagnosis and to potentially treat the fetus at the same time. This is purely a research procedure.

Polycystic kidneys
- Autosomal dominant polycystic kidney disease (ADPKD) is the third most common single cause of end-stage renal failure worldwide and has an incidence of 1:400–1000 live births. It is characterized by multiple cysts in both kidneys, cysts in the liver, seminal vesicles, pancreas and arachnoid membrane, and extrarenal abnormalities such as intracranial aneurysms, dilatation of the aortic root, aortic dissection, mitral valve prolapse, and abdominal wall hernias.

- Disease severity in ADPKD is highly variable, ranging from rare in utero cases with massively enlarged cystic kidneys through more typical presentations with end-stage renal disease in the sixth decade, to cases with satisfactory renal function into old age.

- Autosomal recessive polycystic kidney disease (ARPKD) is much rarer and has an incidence of 1 in 20 000 live births. It is characterized by various combinations of bilateral renal cysts and congenital hepatic fibrosis.

- ADPKD has two disease loci: *PKD1*(chromosome 16) and *PKD2* (chromosome 4). All typical cases of ARPKD are linked to a mutation in a single locus, *PKHD1* (chromosome 6).

- Cysts in ARPKD are derived from collecting ducts, but may arise equally from all segments of the nephron and collecting ducts in the dominant form.

- The proteins encoded by *PKD1* and *PKD2* – polycystin-1 and polycystin-2 – are membrane glycoproteins. The ARPKD locus *PKHD1* encodes fibrocystin. Disruption of these proteins in tubular epithelia causes de-differentiation, excessive fluid secretion, and proliferation leading to cyst development.
- Although both forms of polycystic kidney disease have been reported in the in utero period, ARPKD is more common. The diagnosis should be suspected in patients with a positive family history or when large hyperechogenic kidneys are seen on prenatal ultrasound.
- Oligohydramnios may be gradual and is associated with a poor prognosis. There is no fetal therapy available. Termination of pregnancy is usually offered for severe oligohydramnios/anhydramnios when pulmonary hypoplasia is likely.
- Prenatal counseling with a pediatric nephrologist and fetal medicine specialist is important. The diagnosis is usually made after birth or postmortem. Prenatal diagnosis by CVS or amniocentesis is possible in both forms of the disease. Genetic counseling is essential.
- The recurrence risk of severe, early onset, autosomal dominant polycystic kidney disease in siblings has been estimated to be 25%.

Ovarian cysts
- The etiology of fetal ovarian cysts is unclear but includes follicle stimulation by fetal gonadotrophins, maternal estrogen, and placental chorionic gonadotrophins.
- Maternal risk factors that have been reported include diabetes, Rh isoimmunization, and pre-eclampsia. This may be due to the increase

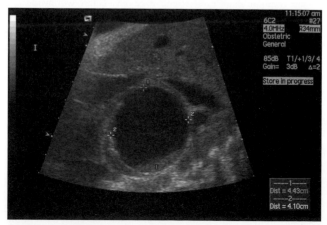

Fig. 8.4. Fetal ovarian cyst.

in maternal gonadotrophin levels associated with these conditions. Fetal hypothyroidism is also reported as a further risk factor.

- Although symptomatic cysts require intervention, simple asymptomatic cysts 4–5 cm in diameter can be managed conservatively (Fig. 8.4). Larger cysts may undergo torsion and intervention is advocated. Most cases of torsion occurs in utero.
- Complex cysts usually represent torsion. Morbidity from untreated torted cysts can be significant, including loss of the ovary, intraperitoneal hemorrhage, peritonitis, and intestinal obstruction.
- Differential diagnoses include mesenteric, omental, or duplication cysts. Ovarian cysts are, however, more lateral and situated low in the pelvis in a female fetus.
- Aspiration may need to be considered if the cyst is >4–5 cm in diameter to prevent torsion. Aspirated cysts have a much higher incidence (>80%) of resolving after birth in contrast to non-aspirated cysts. Intervention is not required if the cyst appears complex on ultrasound.
- After birth, the neonate will require an ultrasound scan to confirm the diagnosis. Most simple ovarian cysts resolve spontaneously; however, a proportion will persist and will require surgery.

8

GENITOURINARY TRACT ABNORMALITIES

9 SKELETAL SYSTEM ABNORMALITIES

- There are more than 200 skeletal dysplasias, a heterogeneous group of genetic disorders characterized by differences in the size, shape, and mineralization of the skeletal system that frequently result in disproportionate short stature. The diagnosis is usually made by clinical features, radiological criteria, family history and, increasingly, by genetic testing.
- It is estimated that 30–45 per 100 000 newborns have a skeletal dysplasia.
- Antenatal management depends on identifying the presence of a skeletal dysplasia and making a assessment of the lethality of the condition.
- Family history of skeletal dysplasia, malformations, and short stature should be obtained.
- Detailed ultrasound is required to evaluate all long bones including pelvic bones for shape, length, and fractures. Mineralization should be assessed qualitatively in the calvarium, ribs, and spine. Skull shape and thoracic cage should be examined.
- Other abnormalities, particularly facial clefts, polydactyly, and talipes should be excluded. If Ellis–van Creveld syndrome is suspected, fetal echocardiography should be performed. Fetal growth restriction should be excluded. Isolated moderate symmetrical limb shortening with structurally intact skeleton is often due to intrauterine growth restriction.
- Karyotyping should be offered particularly in the presence of other abnormalities. DNA should be stored for future genetic testing. A precise diagnosis often needs to await postnatal or postabortal radiology or molecular testing.
- Most cases of skeletal dysplasias are autosomal recessive, for which genetic counseling is important. Others may be due to a new dominant mutation, which may still increase recurrence risks due to gonadal mosaicism.
- Amnioreduction may be required if polyhydramnios is severe (amniotic fluid index (AFI) >40 cm).
- The phenotype of the external genitalia should be confirmed as discordance between karyotype and external genitalia may indicate campomelic dysplasia.
- Termination of pregnancy is an option for most cases of skeletal dysplasias as many have a poor outcome. A narrow thorax (Fig. 9.1), in particular, indicates a high chance of lethal pulmonary hypoplasia.

Achondroplasia
- Achondroplasia is the most common non-lethal skeletal dysplasia and is inherited in an autosomal dominant fashion.
- Clinical findings arise secondary to gain-of-function mutations in the fibroblast growth factor receptor-3 (FGFR3) gene, which has been mapped to chromosome 4p16.3.

9

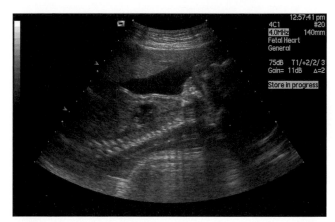

Fig. 9.1. Narrow thorax with hypoplastic lungs.

SKELETAL SYSTEM ABNORMALITIES

- More than 99% of people with achondroplasia carry a point mutation in one copy of the FGFR3 gene. Rare cases of achondroplasia have been attributed to other mutations in FGFR3. Advanced paternal age is associated with an increased incidence of new mutations causing achondroplasia.
- Most cases are due to a sporadic new mutation in the FGFR3 gene.
- Other disorders linked to mutations in FGFR3 include thanatophoric dysplasia (Types I and II), hypochondroplasia, severe achondroplasia with developmental delay, and acanthosis nigricans (SADDAN dysplasia), and two craniosynostosis disorders: Muenke coronal craniosynostosis and Crouzon syndrome with acanthosis nigricans.
- Homozygous achondroplasia (the majority of cases are heterozygous), where individuals have mutations in both of their FGFR3 genes, is neonatally lethal and the skeletal manifestations are of severe achondroplasia – pronounced rhizomelia, marked midface hypoplasia, macrocephaly, very small foramen magnum, and short ribs resulting in a small thorax and restricted respiration. Death usually results secondary to respiratory compromise or from cervical cord compression.
- Most prenatal cases are diagnosed in the third trimester when femur growth falls off significantly (Figs. 9.2 and 9.3). It would be unusual for the diagnosis to be entertained at the routine second trimester fetal anomaly scan. Other long bones will also be similarly short (Figs. 9.4 and 9.5).
- The differential diagnoses include intrauterine growth restriction and hypochondroplasia, although other skeletal dysplasias remain possibilities.

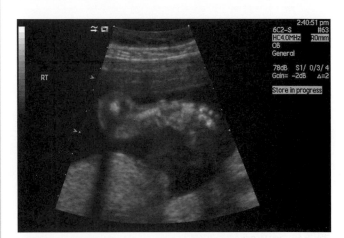

Fig. 9.2. Short humerus.

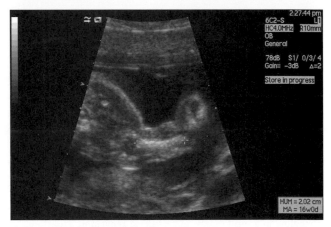

Fig. 9.3. Achondroplasia with short femur.

- If the diagnosis is suspected on ultrasound, karyotyping and FGFR3 testing should be performed. Comprehensive fetal Doppler assessment should be carried out to exclude growth restriction. Genetic counseling should be offered.
- Respiratory problems, tibial bowing, weight gain, and obesity are major problems in achondroplasia and contribute to morbidity associated with spinal stenosis and non-specific joint problems.

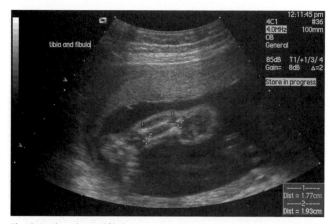

Fig. 9.4. Short tibia and fibula.

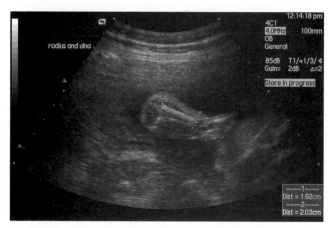

Fig. 9.5. Short radius and ulna.

- Nutritional counseling is advisable to help children with achondroplasia stay within 1 s.d. on height-for-weight curves developed for children with achondroplasia.
- Multidisciplinary follow-up and management are important for children with achondroplasia. Although achondroplasia is not associated with growth hormone deficiency, trials investigating the efficacy of growth hormone therapy in increasing height in achondroplasia have long

been reported. Growth hormone plays an important role in regulating linear skeletal growth by promoting chondrocyte proliferation directly or indirectly through insulin–like growth factor-1.

- The majority of growth hormone trials in children with achondroplasia have been short term with 65%–75% improvement in growth velocity. Long-term efficacy is unclear.

Campomelic dysplasia

- Campomelic dysplasia has an incidence of 1 in 200 000 births and is characterized by symmetrical bowing of the long bones of the lower extremeties, sex reversal in some chromosomally male infants, and other associated structural anomalies (cleft palate, micrognathia, ventriculomegaly, renal abnormalities, and cardiac abnormlities).
- It results from either autosomal dominant inheritance or gonadal mosaicism. Mutations in the *SOX9* gene located at 17q24–q25 locus have been implicated in the etiology. Mutations in *SOX9* have shown an association with both campomelic dysplasia and sex reversal.
- *SOX9* is an SRY-box-containing gene that encodes a transcriptional activator and is essential for diverting an intrinsically ovarian program of organogenesis toward testis formation.
- The main ultrasound features include acute angulation of the junction of the upper and lower thirds of the femur, hypoplastic scapulas, marked micrognathia, mild bilateral hydronephrosis, ventriculomegaly, and talipes. Cardiac abnormalities are present in 25% of cases. Polyhydramnios may be present in a significant proportion of cases.
- If the diagnosis is suspected antenatally, karyotyping is indicated with *SOX9* mutation analysis. The external genitalia should be examined to ascertain any discordance between the observed phenotype and chromosome results.
- The main differential diagnosis is osteogenesis imperfecta Type III because of bowing in the lower limbs. In campomelic dysplasia, tibial bowing is more marked as is the presence of additional anomalies.
- Termination of pregnancy should be discussed and offered.
- There is an increased incidence of stillbirth. The majority of surviving newborns die within the first year of life. Respiratory distress is common and mechanical ventilation usually required. Delivery in a tertiary center is recommended.
- Postdelivery a whole body X-ray will help with the diagnosis. Postmortem should be performed. Genetic counseling is essential.

Diastrophic dysplasia

- Diastrophic dysplasia is a rare skeletal dysplasia associated with severe limb distortion and micromelia, spinal abnormalities, cleft palate, talipes, "hitchhiker thumb," and irregular calcifications of the pinnae of the ears ("cauliflower ears"). It is the most common skeletal dysplasia in Finland.
- The diastrophic dysplasia sulfate transporter (*DTDST*) gene is a novel gene that has been shown to be the cause of the disease. The gene is

found on chromosome 5 and encodes a Na^+-independent membrane transporter of sulfate. High levels of DTDST mRNA are present in human cartilage and intestines. Although the exact function of the gene is unknown, the DTDST-mediated sulfate transport system in chondrocytes may have an important role in endochondral bone formation.

- Intelligence is usually normal and there is a wide variation in the phenotypic abnormalities (cleft palate, scoliosis/lordosis, talipes, ulnar deviation of the hand, limitation of joint movement, shortened first metacarpal ("Hitchhiker's thumb")). Long-term problems are mainly orthopedic in nature.

- If the diagnosis is suspected, karyotyping and genetic testing for mutations in the *DTDST* gene are indicated. Serial scans and genetic counseling are necessary. Termination of pregnancy is an option and should be discussed.

- Diastrophic dysplasia is inherited as an autosomal recessive condition. Mutations in the *DTDST* gene are also responsible for disorders such as atelosteogenesis Type II and achondrogenesis Type IB.

Osteogenesis imperfecta

- Osteogenesis imperfecta is a genetic disorder of increased bone fragility and low bone mass caused by a mutation in one of the two genes that encode procollagen Type1. The severity can vary widely, ranging from intrauterine fractures and perinatal lethality to very mild forms without fractures.

- Associated extraskeletal abnormlities include blue sclera, dentinogenesis imperfecta, hyperlaxity of ligaments and skin, hearing impairment, and presence of wormian bones on skull radiographs.

- The original classification by Sillence in 1979 described four clinically distinct subtypes. Osteogenesis imperfecta Type I includes patients with mild disease. Although vertebral fractures are common and can lead to mild scoliosis, major bone deformities are rare. Type II is lethal in the perinatal period, usually because of respiratory failure resulting from multiple rib fractures. Osteogenesis imperfecta Type III is the most severe form in children surviving the neonatal period. Very short stature, limb and spine deformities, secondary to multiple fractures and respiratory difficulties, are the leading cause of death in this group. Osteogenesis imperfecta Type IV results in mild to moderate bone deformities and variable short stature.

- Hearing impairment is common in Type I disease but rare in Types III and IV.

- The most typical sequence abnormality associated with osteogenesis imperfecta is a point mutation that affects a glycine residue in either *COL1A1* or *COL1A2*. Cells harboring such a mutation produce a mixture of normal and abnormal collagen. Genotype–phenotype correlations are currently unable to predict with certainty the phenotypic effect of a particular glycine mutation.

- Patients with Type I disease secrete half the normal amount of Type I procollagen. Abnormal molecules are not produced in Type I in

9

contrast to the other types in which a mixture of both normal and abnormal Type I procollagen is secreted.

- Ultrasound findings include in utero fractures (long bones and ribs) with callus formation, limb shortening, and poor ossification, particularly of the cranium, resulting in unusual clarity of intracranial structures.

- In the absence of a family history, most antenatally detected cases will be Type II osteogenesis imperfecta.

- Differential diagnoses include other causes of severe skeletal dysplasia and demineralization: hypophosphatasia, achondrogenesis, and campomelic dysplasia. Demineralization is not a typical feature seen in achondrogenesis or campomelic dysplasia.

- If the diagnosis is suspected antenatally, tertiary referral is indicated. Genetic counseling is essential and a family history of blue sclerae, fractures, deafness, and height should be obtained.

- Invasive testing is indicated to obtain samples for *COL1A1* and *COL1A2* mutation analysis. Most prenatally diagnosed cases on ultrasound will be Type II disease with very poor prognosis. Termination of pregnancy should be discussed and offered.

- Caesarean section is generally advisable (for Types I, III and IV), as it minimizes the risk of trauma during delivery. For Type II disease, the perinatal outcome is so poor that vaginal delivery is probably more appropriate, although this should be discussed fully with the patient.

- Most cases are autosomal dominant, the result of a new mutation. Autosomal recessive disease is rare except in consanguineous families. The risk increases with a second affected child, as this suggests that the parents are mosaic carriers of the mutant gene.

- Prenatal diagnosis in subsequent pregnancies is possible by ultrasound, molecular analysis of chorionic villi or amniocytes, or by biochemical analysis of a prenatal sample (particularly if the molecular defect is unknown in the affected family).

Ellis–van Creveld syndrome

- Ellis–van Creveld syndrome (EVC) is a chondroectodermal dysplasia characterized by short ribs, polydactyly, growth restriction, and ectodermal and heart abnormalities (50%–60% of cases). It belongs to the short rib–polydactyly group of skeletal dysplasias.

- It is a rare disease with an incidence of 1 in 60 000 live births and is more common in communities where consanguineous relationships are more prevalent.

- On ultrasound, postaxial polydactyly, cardiac malformations (atrial septal defect (ASD), ventricular septal defect (VSD), single atrium), mild micromelia, and distal shortening of limbs are seen. Narrowing of the thorax is usually mild. Differential diagnoses include Jeune syndrome, McKusick–Kaufman syndrome, Weyers syndrome, and achondroplasia.

- It is inherited as an autosomal recessive trait with variable expression. Mutations of the *EVC1* and *EVC2* genes, on chromosome 4p16, have been identified as causative. The diagnosis is based on clinical findings supported by the skeletal survey. The definitive diagnosis is molecular, based on homozygosity for a mutation in the *EVC1* and *EVC2* genes by direct sequencing.

- Management during the neonatal period mainly involves treatment of respiratory distress due to the narrow chest and heart failure. Long-term prognosis is linked to the respiratory difficulties in the first months of life due to the thoracic narrowing and associated heart defects. Prognosis of the final body height is difficult to predict.
- Genetic counseling is essential. The recurrence risk is 25%.

9

SKELETAL SYSTEM ABNORMALITIES

FETAL TUMORS

Teratoma

- Teratomas are tumors that contain tissue from all three germinal layers (ectodermal, mesodermal, and endodermal tissue). Most prenatally diagnosed teratomas are situated in the brain, oropharynx, sacrococcygeal, mediastinum, abdomen, and gonad.
- They tend to have a disorganized heterogeneous appearance on ultrasound with solid, cystic, or complex components and can be very vascular.
- Teratomas are the most common perinatal tumor, comprising 37%–52% of congenital neoplasms and having a yearly incidence of approximately 1 in 40 000 live births.
- 60% of all teratomas are in the sacrococcygeal region gonads (20%), followed by thoraco-abdominal lesions (15%).
- The majority of teratomas diagnosed prenatally tend to be extragonadal and histologically benign. However, fetal lesions are associated with a high mortality rate, particularly if hydrops or preterm delivery supervenes.

Cervical teratoma

- These are rare tumors with males and female fetuses equally affected.
- They occur in the head and neck region and are irregularly shaped vascular lesions containing solid and cystic components. Large masses can distort the cervical and facial anatomy, making assessment of the fetus difficult. Areas of calcification are present in up to 50% of cases.
- Neural tissue is the predominant histological component for these tumors and maternal serum alphafetoprotein (AFP) levels may be very high.
- Polyhdramnios can complicate up to 40% of cases, particularly if the tumor is very vascular.
- Malignant transformation is extremely rare (<5%) and the risk of malignancy increases the older the patient is at the time of diagnosis.
- Tracheal and esophageal obstruction can lead to acute respiratory failure in the newborn, or to prenatal polyhydramnios.
- Differential diagnoses include cystic hygroma, congenital goiter, solid thyroid tumors, neuroblastoma, hamartoma, hemangioma, or lymphangioma.
- The pregnancy should be managed in a tertiary center. Serial weekly or fortnightly scans are necessary to monitor tumor size, liquor volume and fetal well-being. Fetal echocardiography should be performed. Fetal MRI is of benefit both to assess the size and extension of the lesion and to help with the diagnosis.
- The development of hydrops should be carefully noted. There is a high incidence of preterm rupture of membranes at delivery.
- Management of delivery is critical as many of these tumors are large and vascular and can tear or rupture during delivery. Compression of

10

the fetal airway by the tumor mass can result in immediate and catastrophic respiratory compromise at birth.

- Caesarean section is the preferred mode of delivery with the ex-utero intrapartum treatment (EXIT) procedure reserved for cases where there is a significant risk of upper airway obstruction following delivery. This procedure involves partially delivering the baby, whilst maintaining uteroplacental blood flow and fetal gas exchange by keeping the uterus relaxed with the use of tocolytic agents (mainly inhalational). The umbilical cord is not clamped and the baby remains on uteroplacental bypass, while an attempt is made to secure the airway.

- Definitive management of these tumors is surgical excision. This should be performed soon after birth to obviate the risk of respiratory impairment and prevent less common sequelae (sepsis, ulceration, coagulopathy, and hemodynamic disturbance).

- Surgery to remove these masses is complex and often multiple procedures are required. The operative mortality risk can be as high as 15%. Postsurgery, some infants are at risk of transient or permanent hypothyroidism and hypoparathyroidism. Long-term follow-up to detect recurrence is essential.

FETAL TUMORS

Sacrococcygeal teratoma

- Sacrococcygeal teratomas (SCT) are the most common neoplasm in the fetus and newborn, with an estimated prevalence of 1 in 30 000–40 000. There is a 3:1 female preponderance.

- The diagnosis is often made when a complex mass is detected at the base of the spine (sacrococcygeal region) (Figs. 10.1 and 10.2). The tumor can be either predominantly solid and vascular or predominantly cystic with relatively little vascularity or mixed with equal amounts of solid and cystic structures.

- Staging (Altman staging system) is based on the amount of intrapelvic (presacral) extension and external tumor present. Type I – completely external, Type II – equal external and presacral components, Type III – predominantly presacral component extending into abdomen, Type IV – completely presacral with no external component.

- Associated anomalies are present in 10%–40% of cases.

- SCTs can grow to a massive size sometimes as large as the fetus itself. Arterial–venous shunting through the vascular component of the tumor can result in hydrops, polyhydramnios, and high-output cardiac failure. Poor prognostic factors include large solid tumors (>10 cm), hydrops, and polyhydramnios.

- Other complications include gastrointestinal or bladder outlet obstruction. Oligohydramnios may be present if there is significant lower urinary tract obstruction.

- Differential diagnoses include lumbosacral myelomeningocele, sacral lipoma, hemangioma, harmatoma, neuroblastoma, neurofibroma, etc.

- Most SCTs are histologically benign. Malignancy is more common with solid tumors and in males.

10

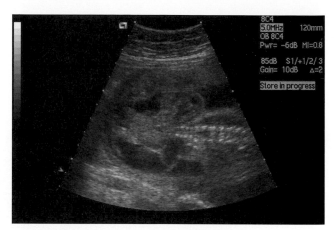

Fig. 10.1. Sacrococcygeal teratoma with solid and cystic elements.

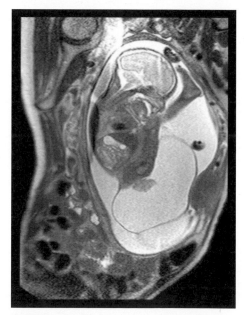

Fig. 10.2. Fetal MRI of sacrococcygeal teratoma.

10

- Tumor dystocia, rupture, and hemorrhage during delivery are the main causes of perinatal morbidity and mortality. Additionally, poly-hydramnios can precipitate preterm delivery (45% risk).
- Maternal complications including pre-eclampsia (Mirror syndrome) can occur if there is significant placentomegaly and hydrops.
- Fetal treatment is possible, mainly for Type I lesions. The criteria for therapy include a large vascular tumour with evidence of hydrops or cardiac overload or polyhydramnios.
- Open fetal surgery has been described but is associated with a significant risk of preterm labor. Less invasive techniques including injection of sclerosants (alcohol) or laser treatment to vaso-occlude the main feeding vessels to the tumor have also been used with success.
- Once a SCT has been identified on antenatal ultrasound, close monitoring is indicated. Large vascular tumors require weekly moni-toring to detect the development of polyhydramnios and/or hydrops. More cystic lesions can be followed up fortnightly.
- Fetal echocardiography is indicated and additional anomalies excluded. Karyotyping is not usually required. Fetal MRI is useful to delineate the extent of intrapelvic/abdominal extension.
- Delivery should take place in a tertiary center with facilities for immediate surgery. Elective Caesarean section should be the mode of delivery, with particular care taken during delivery to avoid trauma to the tumor. Blood should be available in the delivery room in case of tumor hemorrhage.
- If the baby is stable at delivery without evidence of cardiac dysfunction, surgery can take place after further investigations. If a hyperdynamic circulation is present with high-output cardiac failure, surgery becomes more urgent once the baby is stabilized.
- The key factor determining long-term outcome is the age at diagnosis with earlier diagnosis (<2 months) having the lowest risk of long-term malignant sequelae (5%–10%). Recurrence rates range from 2%–35% of patients.
- Recurrence is due to several factors: failure to achieve complete resection of the tumor, tumor spillage, and failure to detect malignant components within the tumor. Most tumors that undergo malignant transformation are Type IV lesions. Good cosmetic outcome is possible in many cases (Figs. 10.3 and 10.4).
- Although the long-term outcome is generally excellent, a significant number of survivors can have functional problems which affect their quality of life. Faecal incontinence (7%), urinary incontinence (30%), constipation (13%), and involuntary bowel movements (9%) can all be long-term issues following surgery.
- Most cases are sporadic and are unlikely to recur.

Wilm's tumor
- Wilm's tumor is a pediatric kidney cancer that affects 1 in 10 000 children. It is the most common malignant renal tumor in children. Wilm's tumors seem to develop from nephrogenic rests, an abnormal

FETAL TUMORS

10

FETAL TUMORS

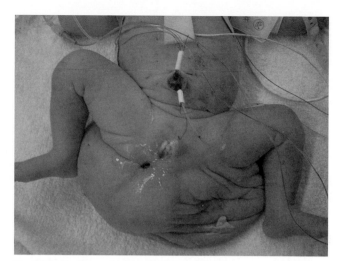

Fig. 10.3. Newborn with large sacrococcygeal teratoma.

structure in the kidney that is formed by failure of the mesenchymal tissue to differentiate into nephrons.

- Additional genetic events are then required to transform these undifferentiated cells, causing uncontrolled growth leading to the formation of massive tumors.

- Homozygous mutations in the Wilm's tumour-suppressor gene *WT1* are found in approximately 18% of Wilm's tumors. *WT1* is required for kidney induction and has an important role in nephron formation and podocyte differentiation. Loss of *WT1* function during kidney development is likely to arrest nephron precursor cells in a multipotent state, making them susceptible to mutations growth-promoting genes.

- The majority of tumors with *WT1* mutations also carry mutations in the β-catenin gene. Although the target genes that are responsible for tumour formation are unknown, β-catenin probably induces the proliferation of precursor cells, leading to cancer.

- A recent discovery is that *WTX*, a novel gene that is mutated in 30% of Wilm's tumors and appears to act as a negative regulator of β-catenin. *WTX* is the first tumor-suppressor gene to be identified that is linked to the X chromosome. Because it lies in a chromosomal region that undergoes X inactivation, both male and females have only one functional copy of this gene and, as a consequence, a "single-hit" mutation is sufficient to result in inactivation.

- Wilm's tumor may be isolated or may occur as part of a genetic syndrome (Beckwith–Wideman, Perlman, neurofibromatosis, Klippel–Trenaunay). Other associated anomalies include aniridia, cryptorchidism,

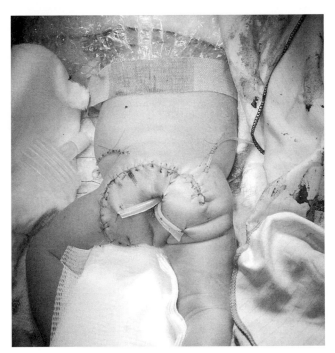

Fig. 10.4. Post-resection of tumor.

hypospadias, and hemihypertrophy and in 5% of cases there is bilateral renal involvement.

- Fetal diagnosis is very rare and the main differential diagnoses of a large renal mass include hydronephrosis, multicystic dysplastic kidney, mesoblastic nephroma, and neuroblastoma.
- Serial scans are necessary to assess growth of the renal mass. Karyotyping and genetic screening may be necessary if a genetic condition is suspected. Fetal MRI may be helpful.
- Delivery should take place in a tertiary center. Further investigations (ultrasound, CT, MRI) to define the mass, as well as to ascertain the presence of metastasis, is required.
- Laparotomy and nephro-ureterectomy and evaluation of the contralateral kidney are required to exclude synchronous lesions. Depending on the stage and histology of the tumor, radiotherapy and chemotherapy may be required.
- The relapse-free survival rate at 2 years now exceeds 90%. Anaplastic lesions have poorer survival rates and represent a therapeutic challenge.

10

- The sporadic form of Wilm's tumor is not associated with recurrence. However, 20% of patients with Wilm's tumor are at risk of recurrence in a sibling.

Liver tumors

- Tumors of the liver are rare during the prenatal and neonatal period. They account for only 5% of all neoplasms that occur in the fetus and the newborn. Common lesions are hemangiomas, mesenchymal hamartomas, and hepatoblastomas. The most common tumor that metastasizes to the liver in the fetus and neonate is neuroblastoma.
- Hemangiomas are usually large, well-defined, echogenic intrahepatic masses, often containing echo-free areas. Arterial venous shunting can occur through a hemangioma, resulting in secondary hydrops.
- Hemangiomas are relatively common, occurring in as many as 1 in 100 neonates. The incidence of mesenchymal hamartomas is uncertain but there is a male preponderance. Hepatoblastomas are the leading primary hepatic malignancy occurring within the first year of life.
- There are five hepatoblastoma histologic subtypes: fetal, embryonal, mixed epithelial, mesenchymal/macrotrabecular, and small cell undifferentiated.
- The fetal subtype carries the most favorable prognosis and small cell undifferentiated the worst. There is an increased incidence of hepatoblastoma in Beckwith–Wiedeman (10%), hemihypertrophy, and familial adenomatous polyposis (FAP).
- Aneuploidy has been associated with hepatoblastoma and karyotyping is therefore indicated if it is suspected prenatally.
- If a liver mass is diagnosed antenatally, color Doppler should be used to differentiate a hemangioma from other tumors. Associated anomalies should be excluded. Organomegaly and macroglossia should be specifically looked for to exclude Beckwith–Wideman syndrome.
- Maternal AFP levels are markedly elevated in cases of hepatoblastoma and mesenchymal harmatoma.
- Mesenchymal hamartoma is more common in the right lobe of the liver. On ultrasonography, multiple echogenic cysts are present or, if the cysts are small, the entire tumor may appear as an echogenic mass.
- Fetal MRI may help delineate the size and extent of the tumor.
- The patient should be managed in a tertiary center with facilities for pediatric surgery. Once delivery has taken place, a definitive diagnosis should be made.
- Hepatic hemangiomas are associated with cutaneous hemangiomas in 50% of cases. Thrombocytopenia may be present. Many of these lesions are discovered incidentally and are localized and small enough to be of no clinical significance.
- A large rapidly growing hemangioma can produce life-threatening complications in the form of intractable high-output cardiac failure from significant arteriovenous shunting, Kasabach–Merritt syndrome,

10

intraperitoneal hemorrhage, and respiratory distress as a result of pulmonary congestion and massive hepatomegaly can occur.

- Kasabach–Merritt syndrome is a localized intravascular coagulopathy associated with profound platelet trapping within the tumor.
- Recent studies have shown that large hemangiomas may produce antibodies to thyroid stimulating hormone (TSH), and screening to rule out secondary hypothyroidism is recommended.
- Treatment of hepatic hemangiomas can involve the use of cortico-steroids, interferon, and embolization. Smaller lesions can be managed expectantly.
- In cases of mesenchymal harmatoma and hepatoblastoma, surgical resection is the treatment of choice. With the addition of platinum-based chemotherapeutic agents, 3-year survival rates for stage 1 hepatoblastomas are now approaching 100%. The long-term outcome for mesenchymal harmatomas following complete excision is excellent.
- Liver transplantation is a good treatment option in children with unresectable primary hepatoblastomas and without demonstrable metastatic disease after neoadjuvant chemotherapy.
- In large solitary, and especially multifocal, hepatoblastomas invading all four sectors of the liver, transplantation has resulted in long-term disease-free survival in up to 80% of children.

FETAL TUMORS

11 FETAL GROWTH ABNORMALITIES

Fetal growth

- Fetal growth and development are complex processes that rely on multiple interacting maternal and uteroplacental factors that ultimately determine the size of the fetus. Both genetic (particularly maternal genes) and environmental factors influence this process.
- Adequate maternal nutrition is essential to ensure appropriate fetal growth. Increased caloric intake in the second and third trimesters is important for both fetal and placental growth. Protein intake appears to be particularly important. A Cochrane systematic review found that balanced protein-energy supplementation was able to reduce the risk of small for gestational age neonates by approximately 30%.
- Glucose is also an important nutrient in the control of fetal growth. Studies in diabetic women have shown that very tight glycemic control results in smaller babies, whereas hyperglycemia increases the risk of macrosomic infants.
- Fetal gender is known to affect fetal growth, with male babies are larger on average than female babies. Smoking reduces birth weight by approximately 150–200 g and produces largely symmetrical growth restriction.
- Altitude is a strong predictor of maternal hypoxia and therefore of fetal size. It's effect is greater on the fetal abdominal circumference rather than on head measurements and mean birth weight can be reduced by as much as 400 g.
- Many auto-immune conditions or other chronic inflammatory diseases can have an adverse effect on fetal growth. A combination of reduced feto-placental blood flow, relative hypoxia, and the presence of pro-inflammatory substances adversely affect fetal growth. Such conditions include pre-eclampsia, infections, systemic lupus erythematosus (SLE), and chronic renal disease.

The placenta and fetal growth

- At term, the total placental surface area for gas and nutrient exchange is almost $11 \, m^2$. In fetal growth restriction, both placental volume and villous surface area are reduced.
- Adequate trophoblast invasion, increase in uteroplacental blood flow, maternal–fetal transfer of glucose, lipids, amino acids, and other macro/micro nutrients and the production, transfer and proper function of various growth regulating hormones are key factors in regulating fetal growth.
- Maintenance of placental function is energy intensive. The placenta consumes as much as 40% of O_2 and 70% of glucose supplied to the uterus.
- In the first half of gestation, the increase in fetal weight is mainly due to placental glucose and amino acid transport and is directed towards skeletal and muscle growth. Essential fatty acids are deposited in the

developing brain and retina and can account for up to 50% of dry brain weight.
- In the second half of pregnancy, increasing subcutaneous fat deposition occurs. There is increasing conversion of glucose into fat, as well as increased utilization of fatty acids. From 32 weeks onwards, fat stores increase from 3.2% of fetal body weight to 16%.
- The third trimester is characterized by longitudinal fetal growth accompanied by accumulation of essential body stores in preparation for extrauterine life.

The IGF (insulin-like growth factors) axis
- IGF-I and IGF-II are polypeptides similar to that of insulin. They induce somatic cell growth and proliferation as well as influence the transport of amino acids and glucose across the placenta. In animal studies, both IGF-I and IGF-II are required for fetal and placental growth. IGFs bind to two different receptors – Type 1 and Type 2 IGF receptor, which have differing affinities for the two hormones.
- Serum concentrations of IGF-I and IGF-II are higher in pregnant compared with non-pregnant women, with concentrations increasing even further by the third trimester.
- Fetal concentrations of IGF-I and IGF-II increase substantially with advancing gestation with the greatest rise in IGF-I. IGF action is modulated by IGF binding proteins (IGFBP) of which there are six. IGFBP-1 is the major regulator of IGF-I during pregnancy and is produced mainly in the decidua. Phosphorylation or proteolysis of IGFBPs are mechanisms responsible for altering the bioavailability of IGFs during pregnancy.
- Pregnancy-associated plasma protein-A (PAPP-A) is secreted by the decidua into the maternal circulation during pregnancy and cleaves IGFBP-4, a potent inhibitor of IGF-I, thereby increasing its concentrations. Low circulating levels of PAPP-A (usually detected on first trimester aneuploidy screening) have been associated with an increased risk of fetal growth restriction.

Fetal response to stress
- Blood flow to the fetal brain, heart, and adrenal glands is maintained or increased when oxygen delivery to the fetus decreases. These organs depend largely on aerobic metabolism to meet energy requirements, and preservation of blood flow during hypoxic stress is an important adaptive mechanism.
- Blood flow to the lower half of the fetus (kidneys, skin, muscle, bone, gastrointestinal tract, and pulmonary bed) all reduce during periods of either acute or chronic stress.
- In late gestation neuro-hormonal mechanisms are activated in response to hypoxia and acidemia. A hypoxic insult late in pregnancy (cord compression, placental abruption) activates chemoreceptors in the carotid and aortic bodies, causing an immediate vagal response with bradycardia, and simultaneous vasoconstriction mediated by the sympathetic nervous system. An endocrine response follows to maintain

vasoconstriction and tachycardia (adrenaline and noradrenaline) and the renin–angiotensin system is activated and renin and angiotensin II levels rise further maintaining vasoconstriction and blood pressure.

- Other hormones that are released include adrenocorticotrophin (ACTH) and vasopressin from the pituitary gland, atrial natriuretic peptide, cortisol, neuropeptide Y, and adrenomodullin.
- Chronic hypoxia causes fetal adaptation towards decreased cellular oxygen demand, reduced fetal growth, and a gradual return of neuro-humoral factors and fetal acid–base status towards normal baseline levels. This adaptation may have long-term consequences with increased risks for metabolic (diabetes, hyperlipidemia) and cardiovascular (hypertension, heart disease) diseases in adulthood.

Intrauterine growth restriction (IUGR)
- Small for gestational age (SGA) infants are defined as those born with a weight <10th percentile for gestational age. Many babies who are born below the 10th percentile are not growth restricted but are constitutionally small.
- Intrauterine growth restriction is always pathological. The incidence of IUGR is between 3% and 5% of all pregnancies, although in some communities the incidence may be much higher. A fetus may be growth restricted even if it is above the 10th percentile in weight if it is substantially smaller than its growth potential would predict. 50% of SGA babies may be growth restricted.
- Fetuses that fail to reach their genetically predetermined growth potential due to IUGR secondary to placental insufficiency are at increased risk for adverse sequelae both in the short and the long term.
- IUGR can be secondary to fetal, maternal, or placental causes. Fetal causes include aneuploidy (trisomy 13, 18, 16, triploidy) and are found in up to 15% of cases. Non-aneuploid genetic syndromes and fetuses with structural malformations are also associated with fetal growth restriction and need detailed genetic evaluation.
- Uniparental disomy (UPD) conditions (Silver–Russell syndrome) can cause significant growth restriction as part of their phenotype.
- Congenital infections (rubella, cytomegalovirus, toxoplasmosis, herpes simplex, varicella) have been associated with IUGR. Perinatal infections are responsible for up to 5% of cases and are not a recurring cause of IUGR.
- Multiple pregnancy accounts for up to 5% of cases. There is a direct correlation with IUGR and with the number of fetuses present. Growth abnormalities are seen in 15%–20% of twin pregnancies.
- Umbilical cord and placental abnormalities are frequently identified in pregnancies complicated by IUGR. Anatomical abnormalities such as a two-vessel cord and gastroschisis are more common.
- Placental infarctions, chronic villitis, and placental mesenchymal dysplasia can cause IUGR, preterm delivery, and intrauterine death. Placental mesenchymal dysplasia is a vascular abnormality, which can predispose to placental thrombosis.

11

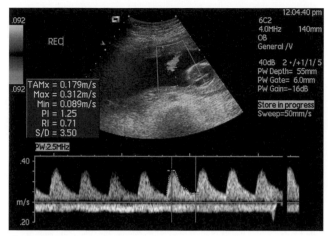

Fig. 11.1. Normal umbilical artery and vein Doppler waveform. See color plate section.

FETAL GROWTH ABNORMALITIES

- Many maternal factors can predispose to IUGR. Cyanotic congenital heart disease, anemia, chronic lung disease, renal failure, hypertension, sickle cell disease, antiphospholipid syndrome, inherited thrombophilias, etc. are all risk factors. Any maternal disease causing vasculopathy (poorly controlled diabetes mellitus, SLE, collagen vascular abnormalities) is a risk factor for IUGR. Early onset preeclampsia is another significant risk factor.
- Recreational drugs (cocaine) and smoking are additional significant risk factors. Smoking may be responsible for up to 20% of cases. Low prepregnancy body mass index (BMI) is also associated with fetal growth restriction.
- Placental dysfunction in IUGR pregnancies can affect the maternal or fetal, or a combination of both vascular beds. Impaired trophoblast invasion and failure of conversion of the maternal spiral arteries can result in abnormal uterine artery Doppler waveforms (notching). If abnormalities occur on the fetal side of the placenta, an increase in umbilical artery Doppler resistance occurs. End–diastolic flow decreases when 30% of the placenta is impaired – this progresses to absent or reversed end-diastolic flow when 60%–70% of the placenta is damaged.
- Assessment and monitoring of the growth–restricted fetus requires comprehensive Doppler analysis of various fetal vessels, liquor volume, and fetal behavior (tone and activity).
- Arterial Doppler waveform analysis provides information on downstream distribution of cardiac output (Fig. 11.1). Venous Dopplers are determined by cardiac compliance, contractility, and afterload and are characterized by a triphasic flow pattern (Fig. 11.2).

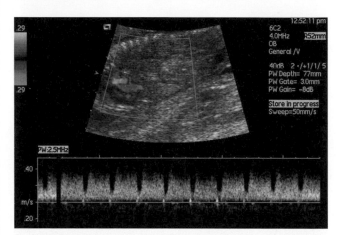

Fig. 11.2. Normal ductus venosus Doppler waveform. See color plate section.

- Forward flow during atrial systole (a-wave) can vary depending on the vein examined. In the inferior vena cava reversal of the "a" wave is physiological. Reversal in the ductus venosus is always pathological.
- Fetal behavioral responses are related to the gestational age and maturity of the central nervous system.
- Compensatory changes in the fetal cardiovascular system and behavioral changes demonstrate a fairly predictable progression. Elevation of the umbilical artery (UA) Doppler index, redistribution of blood flow, and/or brain sparing are early Doppler signs evident before biophysical and fetal heart rate abnormalities occur.
- Progressive fetal compromise results in absent, or reversed umbilical artery end–diastolic flow (EDF) and venous Doppler abnormalities. A decline in amniotic fluid volume may occur concurrently or may precede Doppler abnormalities. Absent or reversed "a" wave in the ductus venosus and cessation of movement and tone are associated with acidemia and a significant risk for stillbirth and neonatal complications.
- With mild placental insufficiency, umbilical and middle cerebral artery Doppler changes may be subtle. With increasing severity, fetal growth velocity decreases and is accompanied by elevation in umbilical artery resistance. Middle cerebral artery impedance (Fig. 11.3) and amniotic volume decreases. Fetal heart rate reactivity may also be lost.
- Once the nadir of cerebral blood flow resistance is reached, aortic blood flow impedance increases. Worsening disease and fetal decompensation result in venous Doppler abnormalities that are inversely correlated with fetal heart rate variability. Absent end–diastolic flow in the umbilical artery is characteristic at this stage.

11

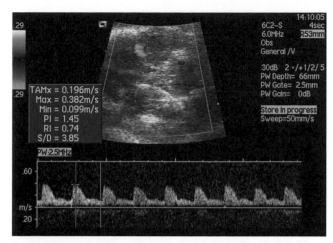

Fig. 11.3. Middle cerebral artery waveform with low pulsatility and resistance indices. See color plate section.

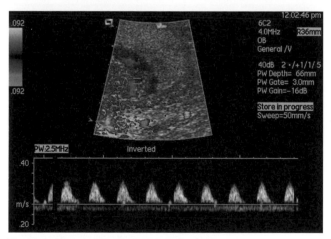

Fig. 11.4. Absent end-diastolic flow. See color plate section.

- With chronic and severe hypoxemia, global fetal activity diminishes and breathing movements cease. Further deterioration of the fetal condition results in reversed umbilical artery end–diastolic velocity and grossly abnormal venous Doppler indices (Figs. 11.4, 11.5, 11.6, and 11.7).

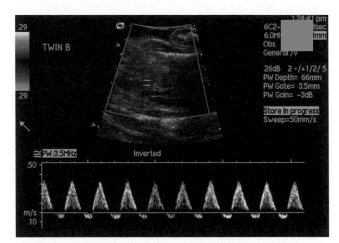

Fig. 11.5. Reverse end-distolic flow. See color plate section.

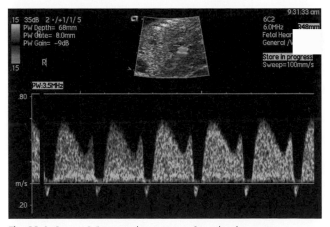

Fig. 11.6. Reverse "a" wave in ductus venosus. See color plate section.

- Pre-terminal events include dilatation of the heart, tricuspid regurgitation, coronary artery dilatation, and spontaneous episodes of bradycardia.
- Brain sparing in the presence of normal venous Doppler parameters identifies IUGR fetuses at risk for hypoxemia. Elevation of venous Doppler indices, either alone, or in combination with a pulsatile umbilical vein, increases the risk for fetal acidemia.

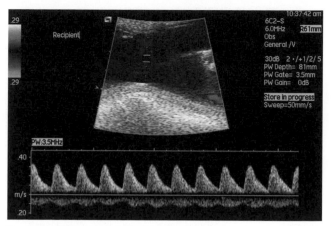

Fig. 11.7. Pulsatile umbilical vein. See color plate section.

- A biophysical profile score of <4 is associated with a mean pH <7.20. A score of <2 has a sensitivity of 100% for the prediction of acidemia. A combination of multivessel Doppler assessment and biophysical profile is probably best used to evaluate the growth-restricted fetus.
- Abnormal venous Doppler parameters are the strongest predictors of stillbirth. The likelihood of stillbirth increases with the degree of venous Doppler abnormality (absent or reversed "a" wave in the ductus venosus and/or umbilical venous pulsations). Abnormalities of venous Doppler indices are associated with a significant increase (11×) in major neonatal complications including neonatal death.
- Neonatal mortality is determined by many factors including gestational age and the severity of neonatal complications. In fetuses with absent or reversed end-diastolic flow (with normal venous indices) rates of 5%–18% have been reported.
- The only therapeutic intervention in IUGR pregnancies is delivery, which is critically influenced by gestational age. Indications for delivery should be based on evidence of fetal compromise from several modalities. Abnormal venous Dopplers with an abnormal biophysical profile score indicates severe fetal compromise indicating delivery.
- There is no good evidence that the intrauterine "stress" of growth restricted fetuses confers a survival benefit over their appropriately grown counterparts.
- Uterine artery Doppler waveform analysis has been used as a screening test for high-risk pregnancies. Bilateral diastolic notching and a mean resistance index of >90th centile at 23 weeks has a positive predictive value of 57% for severe pre-eclampsia +/− IUGR

FETAL GROWTH ABNORMALITIES

11

and a 93% positive predictive value for mild or severe disease. Even in women on low-dose aspirin therapy (because of previous adverse outcome), the presence of a diastolic notch at 23 weeks' gestation is associated with a higher rate (31% vs. 5%) of complications such as pre-eclampsia and IUGR.

- There may be a modest benefit of low-dose aspirin use in pregnancies at high risk for IUGR. A meta-analysis of low-dose aspirin use suggested an 18% reduction in IUGR, but a much greater effect (OR 0.35) when therapy was started before 17 weeks' gestation.
- Aspirin has been found to be especially beneficial in patients with a history of recurrent IUGR, reducing the incidence of fetal growth restriction from 61% in the untreated to 13% in treated pregnancies.
- Depending on the severity of the fetal condition, consideration should be given to referring the patient to a tertiary fetal medicine center so that a comprehensive multi-vessel Doppler assessment of the fetus can be made.
- As there is no fetal intervention to improve outcome, the key decision will be timing of delivery so that complications related to prematurity are minimized and balanced against leaving the fetus in a harsh intrauterine environment.
- Karyotyping should be considered if structural abnormalities present or if early onset growth restriction. Maternal viral serology should also be tested.
- After 32 weeks, delivery is generally indicated once maternal steroids have been administered. Prior to this gestation, monitoring may have to take place very frequently (sometimes even on a daily basis) to enable appropriate timing of delivery.
- Parents should be counseled about the risks (both antenatal and in the neonatal period) to the baby as well as longer-term complications. In cases of severe early-onset growth restriction, termination of pregnancy is an option.
- As many of these babies tolerate the stress of labor poorly, Caesarean section is the usual mode of delivery.
- Full thrombophilia and antiphospholipid screening should be performed after the pregnancy. Selected cases may benefit from aspirin (and heparin).

ABNORMALITIES OF THE EXTREMITIES

Talipes

- Congenital talipes equinovarus (CTEV) is a structural deformity of the lower leg characterized clinically by a combination of a high heel (equinus) and inward tilting of the hindfoot (varus) (Fig. 12.1). The anatomical abnormalities in the limb include malposition of the tarsal bones, atrophy of the calf muscle, and shortness of the foot and limb.

- The etiology is unclear. However, there appears to be a fairly strong genetic component. The mode of inheritance does not follow a clear pattern. Various theories have been proposed, including vascular, viral, genetic, anatomical, following a compartment syndrome, environmental factors, and fetal position in utero. There is still uncertainty whether or not there is a neuromuscular basis for this disorder.

- CTEV occurs in 1.2 per 1000 live births in Europe and is twice as common in boys. First-degree relatives are at a significantly increased risk compared with the general population. A sibling of a patient has a 2% to 4% chance of having CTEV. If a child and another family member, or both parents, have clubfoot, the risk in another child increases by 10%–20%.

- In approximately 20% of cases, CTEV is associated with other congenital abnormalities. Spina bifida is present in approximately 4% of children with talipes, arthrogryposis in 1%, and other various neuromuscular defects in 8%.

- A recent study found that the diagnosis of clubfoot by ultrasound had a positive predictive value of 83% with a false-positive rate of 17%. The false-positive rate appears to be higher for unilateral compared with bilateral abnormalities.

- Once talipes has been detected, careful evaluation of the fetus is necessary to detect additional anomalies. In particular, the attitude of the fetus, abnormalities in other joints, and movement needs to be assessed. Spina bifida should be excluded. Amniotic fluid volume should be measured and serial scans arranged. An assessment of the degree of severity should be made, although there is poor correlation between antenatal diagnosis of severity and the need for further treatment after birth.

- Karyotyping should be considered if additional structural anomalies are present. Genetic referral should also be considered if a neuromuscular diagnosis is a possibility.

- Ideally, the parents should be given the opportunity to meet a pediatric orthopedic surgeon to discuss management antenatally.

- Treatment options (depending on severity) include physiotherapy (continuous passive movement, Bensahel/Dimeglio regime), or surgery. There are various techniques described (Ponseti regime, Ilizarov technique).

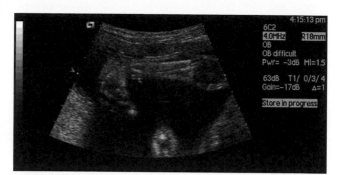

Fig. 12.1. Talipes.

- The Ponseti regime has very good success rates. It involves serial casting of the lower limb using a strictly defined technique. Once the foot is corrected, an abduction foot orthosis must be worn full time initially for 12 hours then at night and at nap time, up to the age of 4 years. Percutaneous tenotomy of the Achillis tendon and transfer of the tibialis anterior tendon are integral parts of the protocol.

- In a recent study, correction of the deformity was obtained in 98% of patients. Minor complications from the cast were encountered in 8% of patients, and 2.5% required extensive corrective surgery. The rate of relapse after initial successful treatment was 10%.

- Bensahel/Dimeglio regime requires daily manipulations of the newborn's clubfeet by a skilled physiotherapist and temporary immobilization with elastic and non–elastic adhesive taping. Most of the improvement occurs in the first 3 months of treatment.

Upper-limb abnormalities

- Congenital anomalies affect 1%–2% of newborns, and approximately 10% of those children have upper-extremity abnormalities.

- Development of the upper extremity commences with formation of the upper-limb bud on the lateral wall of the embryo 4 weeks after fertilization. Eight weeks after fertilization, embryogenesis is complete and all limb structures are present. The majority of congenital anomalies of the upper extremity occur during this period of rapid limb development.

- Various systems exist for the classification of upper-limb malformations on the basis of anatomy, embryology, genetics, and teratology. In utero, fetal hand malformations can be subdivided into (a) alignment abnormalities (clenched hand, camptodactyly, clinodactyly, hypokinesia, clubhand, phocomelia), (b) abnormal thumb, (c) abnormal size (macrodactyly, trident hand), (d) abnormal echogenicity (calcifications), (e) abnormal number of digits (polydactyly, syndactyly, ectrodactyly), and (f) constriction band sequence.

- Many upper-limb abnormalities can be associated with genetic syndromes or other structural anomalies, and careful evaluation of the fetus is essential.

Radial aplasia/hypoplasia

- This affects the preaxial border of the upper limb and can result in a radial club hand. The degree of preaxial deficiency can range from mild thumb hypoplasia to complete absence of the radius. Irrespective of the degree of severity, all forms warrant systemic evaluation for syndromes or associations: Holt–Oram syndrome, thrombocytopenia-absent-radius (TAR) syndrome, VACTERL association (vertebral abnormalities, anal atresia, cardiac abnormalities, tracheoesophageal fistula, esophageal atresia, renal defects, radial dysplasia, and lower-limb abnormalities), and Fanconi anemia are the main differentials.
- Because of the association with other organ systems, fetal echocardiography, assessment of the kidneys and spine, and karyotyping are essential.
- Fanconi's anemia is an aplastic anemia that tends to manifest at a median age of 7 years. Children with Fanconi's anemia do not have signs of bone-marrow failure at birth, and the diagnosis is not apparent initially. The majority of children experience symptoms between the ages of 3 and 12 years. Prenatal diagnosis is possible. Chromosomes isolated from a fetal sample (amniocytes, chorionic villi, fetal blood) treated with di-epoxybutane or mitomycin C, cause chromosome breaks and rearrangements. In contrast, chromosomes from unaffected fetuses are stable when treated with these agents. Bone-marrow transplantation is the only cure for Fanconi anemia.
- If the diagnosis is made prenatally, all options should be discussed including termination of pregnancy.

Ulnar hypoplasia/aplasia

- Ulnar deficiency is four to ten times less common than radial deficiency. It affects the postaxial border of the limb and can be confused with radial deficiency by a sonographer who is not familiar with upper-extremity congenital anomalies. Unlike radial deficiencies, ulnar deficiencies are usually not associated with systemic conditions, but can be related to other musculoskeletal abnormalities.
- The remaining radius assumes characteristics similar to an ulna and can be fused with the distal part of the humerus (radiohumeral fusion). This prevents identification of the proximal part of the radius and results in a bone that resembles an ulna. In addition, the hand can also have radial-sided anomalies ranging from a narrow web space to an absent thumb. Serial evaluations are occasionally necessary in equivocal cases.

Ectrodactyly (cleft hand)

- Split or cleft hand (also known as lobster claw hand) results from a longitudinal deficiency of the central digits. It is caused by probable failure of the median apical ectodermal ridge in the developing limb bud. It has an incidence of 1 in 90 000 live births.

- The malformation is characterized by a deep V- or U-shaped central defect. It may be associated with syndactyly, aplasia, or hypoplasia of the residual phalanges and metacarpals. Hands and feet can be affected (split hand and foot malformation). The severity can be highly variable. Ectrodactyly may be isolated or associated with various autosomal dominant syndromes such as EEC syndrome (ectrodactyly, ectodermal dysplasia, and deft lip or palate), EE syndrome (ectrodactyly and ectodermal dysplasia), Roberts syndrome and LADD syndrome (lacrimo-auriculo-dental-digital). Autosomal recessive and X-linked conditions have also have been described.
- Sonographic findings are the characteristic absence of central digits in the hand. Associated anomalies include cleft lip and palate and genitourinary tract abnormalities.
- Karyotyping should be offered as some conditions are associated with abnormalities on chromosomes 3 and 7. Genetic counseling is essential.
- Once the diagnosis is suspected, referral to a fetal medicine unit is indicated. In addition to genetic counseling, pediatric orthopedic review is also helpful to counsel parents about surgery, the aim of which is to establish opposition between two digits.
- Long-term outcome will depend on the severity of associated abnormalities (sensorineural hearing loss, repeated eye infections, urogenital problems, feeding difficulties, etc.).
- The mode of delivery is made on standard obstetric grounds.

Syndactyly

- Syndactyly is defined as an abnormal interconnection between adjacent digits. The interconnection may encompass the entire length of the adjacent digits (complete) or it may discontinue proximal to the fingertip (incomplete). It may involve only skin and fibrous tissue (simple) or include bone (complex).
- It is a relatively common condition with an incidence of 2–3 per 10 000 and tends to cluster in families. It can also be sporadic or associated with other abnormalities. Familial syndactyly usually affects the second and third digits and is not associated with other abnormalities; transmission is autosomal dominant, with variable expressivity and incomplete penetrance. Associated or complicated syndactyly can be syndromic or secondary to a constriction band sequence. Syndromes described in association with complicated syndactyly include acrocephalosyndactylies and the Poland sequence, and Apert's syndrome. Other associated conditions include Fraser syndrome, Smith–Lemli–Opitz syndrome, and triploidy.
- The diagnosis is often difficult to make on ultrasound but, if detected, careful evaluation of the fetus is essential to detect additional anomalies. Many of the syndromes associated with syndactyly have synostosis of the cranial sutures. This may result in acrocephaly (tall peaked skull with high forehead and frontal bossing).

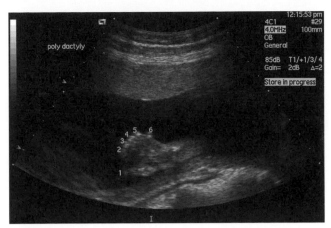

Fig. 12.2. Polydactyly of the hand.

- Careful assessment of the fetus for additional anomalies is essential. Karyotyping is indicated if multiple anomalies are present. Apert's syndrome is associated with mutations in the fibroblast growth factor receptor 2 gene (FGFR2) allowing prenatal diagnosis. Carpenter and Fraser syndromes have a 25% risk of recurrence.
- Genetic counseling is essential once a syndromic diagnosis is made.
- The baby should be seen by a hand surgeon for evaluation of surgery.

Polydactyly
- Polydactyly (extra digits) (Fig. 12.2) can either be on the preaxial (radial) or postaxial (ulnar) side of the limb. Preaxial polydactyly is more common in White people, and postaxial polydactyly is more common in Black people. Postaxial polydactyly in a White individual is rare and may be indicative of an underlying syndrome (e.g. chondroectodermal dysplasia or Ellis–van Creveld syndrome).
- Polysyndactyly corresponds to the association of polydactyly with syndactyly. Polydactyly is one of the most common hand anomalies and is seen in approximately 1 in 700 pregnancies.
- Postaxial polydactyly can be associated with various syndromes: trisomy 13, Meckel–Gruber syndrome (multicystic dysplastic kidneys and posterior encephalocele), Bardet–Biedl syndrome (medullary cystic kidney disease), Smith–Lemli–Opitz syndrome (intrauterine growth retardation and a characteristic high level of 7-dehydrocholesterol), short ribs – polydactyly syndromes (narrow thorax and short ribs), and Ellis–van Creveld syndrome (chondroectodermal dysplasia associated with short ribs, mesomelic shortening of long bones, and cardiac defects).
- Preaxial polydactyly is less commonly seen. If associated with a triphalangeal thumb present, a syndromic diagnosis is likely.

12

ABNORMALITIES OF THE EXTREMITIES

Holt–Oram syndrome (atrial and ventricular septal defects, abnormal thumb – absent or triphalangeal, short ribs – polydactyly syndromes, Carpenter syndrome, trisomy 21, VACTERL association, and Fanconi anemia can all be associated with preaxial polydactyly.

- Once detected, the presence of additional anomalies should be excluded. It is often possible to miss a rudimentary extra digit, particularly if it does not contain bone. If multiple abnormalities are present, aneuploidy is the most likely diagnosis. Karyotyping and DNA analysis may be indicated.
- Genetic counseling is essential if a genetic syndrome is diagnosed. The recurrence risk for isolated familial polydactyly is 50%, and the recurrence risk for other associated conditions or syndromes depends on the specific condition.
- After birth, the baby should be referred to a hand surgeon for further management. The goal of surgery is to achieve optimal function and good cosmetic appearance.

Clinodactyly

- Clinodactyly typically affects the middle phalanx of the small finger and produces an angulation of the distal interphalangeal joint, resulting in a radial deviation. A deviation of $<10°$ is common, and it may be considered normal. Clinodactyly can involve several digits and is usually related to one or more delta-shaped middle phalanges. The deformity is usually fixed with no intra-articular or periarticular swelling.
- It may be isolated or associated with aneuploidy or genetic syndromes. 60% of neonates with Down syndrome have clinodactyly.
- Clinodactyly may result as a consequence of delayed development of the middle phalanx of the little finger.
- Clinodactyly can be inherited and is considered to be an autosomal dominant trait with variable expressivity and incomplete penetrance. Familial clinodactyly is usually not associated with systemic conditions. It may be a feature of several genetic syndromes (Russell–Silver, Cornelia de Lange, Klinefelter, Prader–Willi, Rubenstein–Taybi).
- Karyotyping is not indicated unless additional anomalies are present.
- No specific treatment is required after birth. The long-term cosmetic and functional outcome is excellent.

Transverse limb defects

- Congenital transverse deficiency is defined according to the last remaining bone segment. A short below-the-elbow amputation is the most common transverse deficiency of the upper extremity. There are usually rudimentary nubbins or dimpling on the ends of the affected limb. These abnormalities are usually unilateral, sporadic in occurrence, and rarely associated with other conditions.
- Although limb and digit amputation can occur as a result of amniotic bands (constriction band syndrome), which is the result of entrapment of the developing limb by an amniotic band, the diagnosis of

12

amniotic disruption sequence requires the presence of a constriction band either affecting the involved extremity or elsewhere.

- A less common level of transverse deficiency is through the hand or metacarpals.
- Phocomelia represents a longitudinal failure of formation with an absent intervening segment of the extremity (intercalary aplasia). The missing segment can be the arm or forearm, or both, with the hand attached directly to the shoulder. This deformity is very uncommon but was strongly associated (60%) with maternal ingestion of thalidomide during the first trimester of pregnancy.

Amniotic band syndrome
- Amniotic band syndrome (ABS) is a term applied to a wide range of congenital anomalies, typically limb and digital amputations and constriction rings that occur in association with fibrous bands.
- There are two main theories for the pathogenesis of ABS, and these are referred to as the "extrinsic model" and the "intrinsic model." The intrinsic model (proposed by Streeter in 1930) suggests that the anomalies and the fibrous bands have a common origin, caused by a perturbation of developing germinal disc of the early embryo. Torpin in 1965 proposed what later became the "extrinsic theory," in that the birth defects are caused by the action of the fibrous amniotic bands.
- The extrinsic theory suggests that rupture of the amnion is followed by loss of amniotic fluid and extrusion of all, or parts, of the fetus into the chorionic cavity. The trapped fetus is subjected to compression from the limited space, and the limbs and other body parts become entangled in the shriveled, rolled remnants of amnion.
- The gestational age at which the amniotic sac ruptures is believed to be the major determining factor in influencing the range and severity of abnormalities seen. Early rupture (before day 45 of gestation) is associated with multiple severe deformities which include: scalp and skull vault deficiencies, encephalocoeles, facial clefts, abdominal and thoracic defects, major spinal anomalies, auto-amputations, and intrauterine death. Late rupture of the amnion (after day 45 of gestation) tends to produce limb constrictions.
- Limb–body wall complex syndrome is a major malformation characterized by a anterolateral body wall defect with herniation of abdominal and/or thoracic viscera, short umbilical cord, severe spinal abnormalities including scoliosis, and very close attachment of the fetus to the placenta.
- ABS may also result in simple amputation of digits in the hand and/or feet to more major amputations involving part or most of a limb. Deformities of the skull (encephaloceles) are also common. Constricted limbs may become edematous initially before atrophying. This can sometimes be detected on ultrasound.
- Occasionally, amniotic bands can result from intrauterine instrumentation (amniocentesis) or infection, but this is rare. It has also been reported with genetic syndromes (Ehlers–Danlos Type III and osteogenesis imperfecta).

12

- If limb defects are detected on ultrasound, careful examination for the presence of amniotic bands should be performed. Antenatal referral to a pediatric orthopedic or plastic surgeon for counseling is of benefit.
- Incidentally, detected amniotic bands do not require any treatment if there is no limb entrapment. Serial scans to ensure that the fetus is moving freely in the amniotic cavity may be useful. If there is limb entrapment with a significant risk of distal ischemia and loss in utero, treatment may be considered. Fetoscopic or ultrasound guided division of bands has been described. Karyotyping is not indicated.
- If limb–body wall complex anomaly or any other major structural malformation (encephalocele) is detected, termination of pregnancy should be offered.
- Mode of delivery is made on standard obstetric grounds. In severe cases delivery should take place in a tertiary center with facilities for pediatric orthopedic, and plastic surgery.
- Most cases are sporadic with no risk of recurrence.

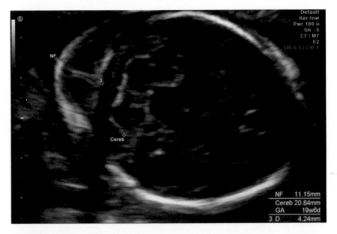

Fig. 2.7. Mid trimester nuchal edema.

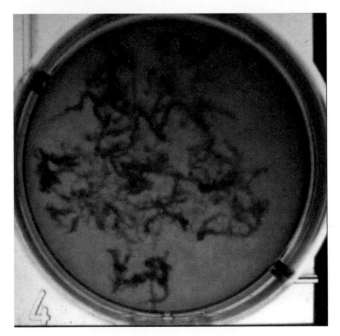

Fig. 3.2. CVS sample.

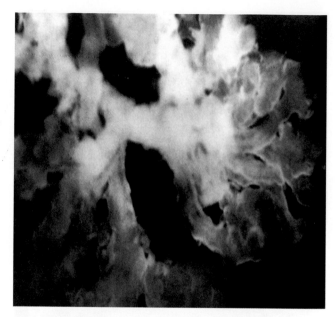

Fig. 3.3. Chorionic villi.

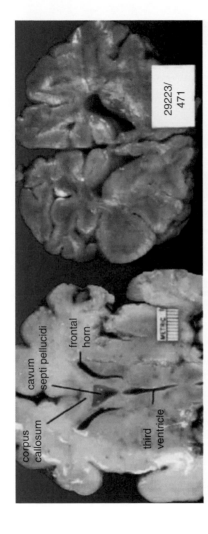

Fig. 4.1. Pathology specimen demonstrating normal brain and agenesis of the corpus callosum.

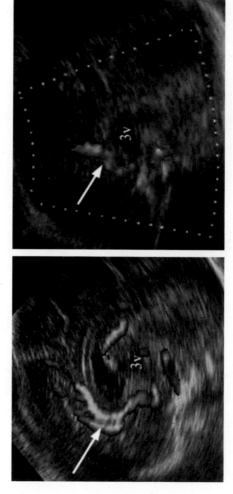

Fig. 4.3. Pericallosal artery.

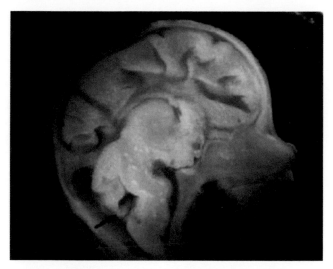

Fig. 4.6. Pathology specimen demonstrating cerebellar vermis hypoplasia.

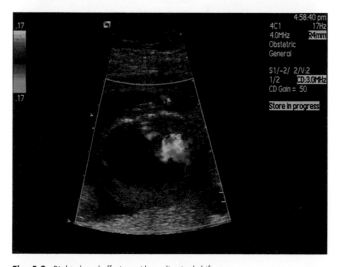

Fig. 5.3. Right pleural effusion with mediastinal shift.

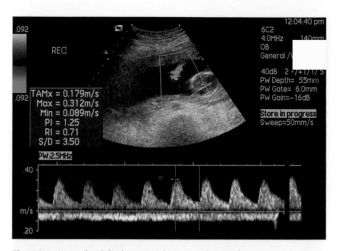

Fig. 11.1. Normal umbilical artery and vein Doppler waveform.

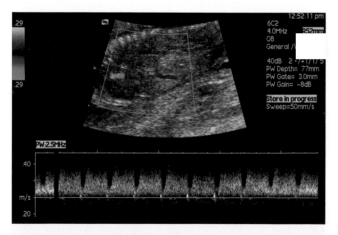

Fig. 11.2. Normal ductus venosus Doppler waveform.

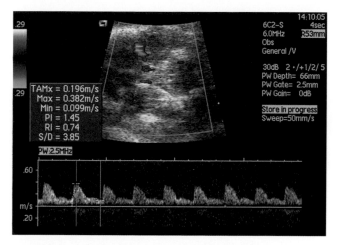

Fig. 11.3. Middle cerebral artery waveform with low pulsatility and resistance indices.

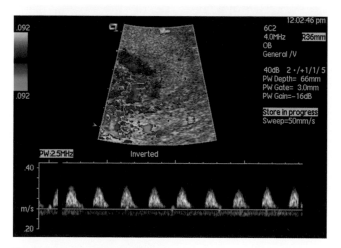

Fig. 11.4. Absent end-diastolic flow.

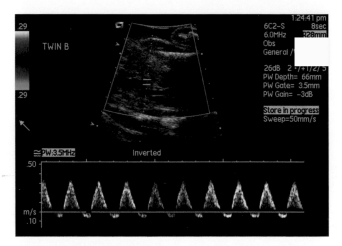

Fig. 11.5. Reverse end-diastolic flow.

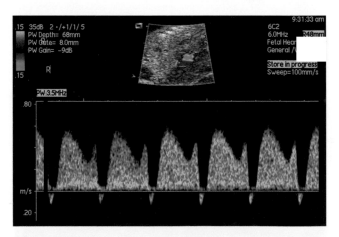

Fig. 11.6. Reverse "a" wave in ductus venosus.

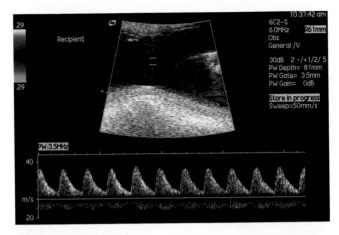

Fig. 11.7. Pulsatile umbilical vein.

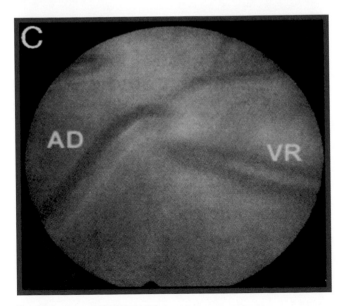

Fig. 15.1. Artery-to-vein anastomosis.

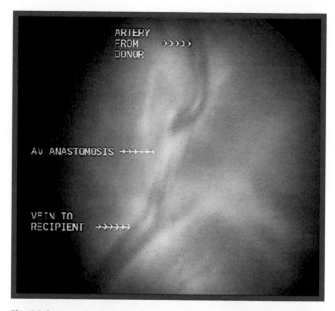

Fig. 15.2. Artery to vein anastomosis on chorionic plate.

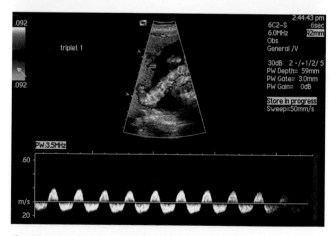

Fig. 15.5. Doppler waveform of an artery-to-artery anastomosis.

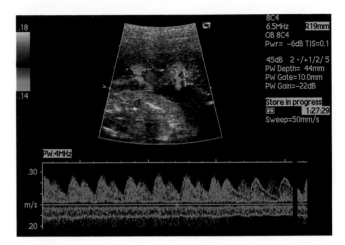

Fig. 15.6. Doppler waveform of cord entanglement showing two asynchronous arterial waveforms.

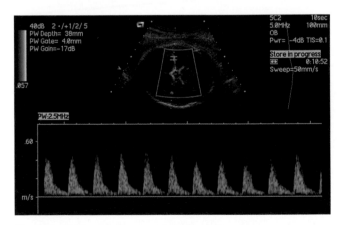

Fig. 18.1. Middle cerebral artery peak systolic velocity.

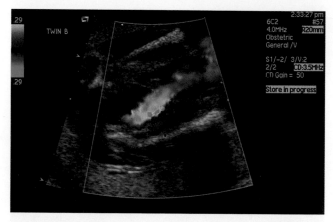

Fig. 19.1. Single umbilical artery.

Cleft lip and palate

- Virtually all cases of cleft lip–cleft palate (CLP) are attributable to the failure of the medial nasal process either to contact or to maintain contact with the lateral nasal and maxillary processes.
- By the end of the eighth week, the face assumes most of the characteristics that make it recognizable as human. The face is derived from five facial prominences that surround the future mouth: single frontonasal process and the paired maxillary and mandibular processes.
- The grooves between these facial prominences usually disappear by day 46 or 47 of gestation, as the processes meet their equivalents from the contralateral side and fuse in the midline. Any persisting groove between meeting or adjoining processes results in a congenital facial cleft.
- The incidence of cleft lip and palate varies with ethnicity and geographical region but in a caucasion population it is approximately 1 in 800–1000 for CLP and 1 in 100 for cleft palate.
- Orofacial clefts can be classified as non-syndromic (isolated) or syndromic based on the presence of other congenital anomalies. Approximately 20%–50% of all orofacial clefts are associated with one of more than 400 described syndromes.
- The cause of CLP is complex and multifactorial, involving both genetic and environmental factors.
- In a family with a CLP child, the chance that a second child will be born with a similar defect is 3%–4%; if two children have the defect, the chance of a third child being born with the defect is 9% and 17%–20% if either parents affected. Recurrence risk of CLP is 50% if any family members have van der Woude syndrome.
- Many environmental factors are associated with orofacial clefting. Maternal alcohol consumption during pregnancy increases the incidence of both syndromic and non-syndromic clefts. Maternal cigarette smoking and orofacial clefting is well established, with at least a doubling of the incidence of CLP compared with non-smoking mothers.
- The effect of maternal smoking appears to be related to increased serum carbon monoxide levels, which exert their effect on cytochrome oxidase.
- Folate deficiency is associated with CLP and prenatal folic acid supplementation has been shown to decrease this risk. Conversely, folic acid antagonists increase the incidence of orofacial clefting.
- Poor nutrition may be a reason for the higher incidence of unusual orofacial clefts found in developing countries.
- Maternal corticosteroid use causes a threefold to fourfold increase in orofacial clefting. Anticonvulsants, including phenytoin and valproic

13

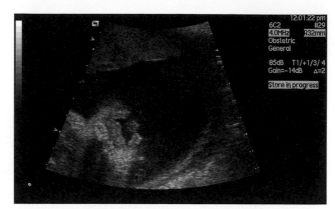

Fig. 13.1. Bilateral cleft lip and palate.

acid also cause cleft lip and palate. Phenytoin causes a nearly tenfold increase in the incidence of facial clefting and exerts its effect by inhibiting enzymes in the NADH dehydrogenase pathway. Other agents including retinoic acid have also been implicated in orofacial clefting, but the exact mechanism of action is unclear.

- Most facial clefts are diagnosed on routine anomaly scan. It is important to obtain a detailed history, particularly of a family history of cleft lip/palate, history of drug exposure, anticonvulsants, alcohol, smoking, or steroids.
- A detailed scan is needed to determine if unilateral/bilateral, and for other structural anomalies and soft tissue markers. Cleft lips are optimally seen in the coronal view (Figs. 13.1 and 13.2). The palate can be visualized by rotating to the axial plane, but is visualized better on 3D scanning. 80% of CLP and 85% of bilateral are isolated.
- 70% of unilateral cleft lip is found in combination with cleft palate. Isolated cleft palate is different genetically from CLP and can be difficult to identify in the presence of an intact lip; a parasagittal view of the fetal face may help.
- Associated anomalies include CNS, cardiac (24%) and limb/spine (33%) deformities. There is a high risk of cerebral anomaly with midline CLP. If views are suboptimal due to fetal position, then a repeat visit may be required. If they remain poor, consider embryo-fetoscopy.
- Karyotyping should be offered in all cases. Risk varies with CLP type: unilateral cleft lip 5%, unilateral CLP 10%, bilateral CLP 20%–30%, midline CLP 50%–80%.
- Counseling will depend on whether CLP is isolated or associated with structural or chromosomal anomalies, whether there is a cleft lip, palate, or both, and whether the cleft is unilateral, bilateral, or midline.

13

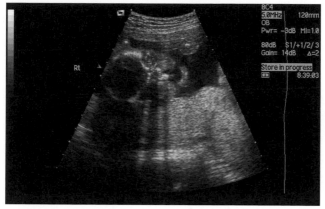

Fig. 13.2. Large bilateral cleft lip.

- Parents should be advised that, even with an apparently isolated CLP, there is a 5%–10% risk of an underlying genetic condition or syndrome.
- Outline postnatal management of the baby. Mention feeding, nipple guards, special bottles, and teats. Surgical correction is usually deferred to 3–6 months for cleft lip and palate, respectively, although lip surgery is increasingly brought forward to the neonatal period.
- Mention ancillary services such as speech therapy and orthodontic treatment. Recommend the Cleft Lip and Palate Association for further advice and information.
- Refer to the multidisciplinary craniofacial team following fetal diagnosis, where all aspects of management including feeding, surgery, and cosmetic results can be discussed with parents.
- Termination of pregnancy may be offered in the presence of aneuploidy or other structural anomalies.
- If the pregnancy is on-going, a repeat scan should be performed at 28–32 weeks to detect any evolving or missed structural anomalies.
- Genetic counseling for the risk of recurrence should be offered, and referral is advised for all but isolated CLP.
- Recurrence risks may be modified by: preconception high dose folic acid (5 mg/day), decreasing or avoiding alcohol, and changing or stopping anticonvulsant drugs (needs discussion with obstetric physician).

Micrognathia
- This is characterized by mandibular hypoplasia and a small receding chin that results in posterior displacement of the base of the tongue into the oropharynx.

13

- Management of children with micrognathia is difficult because of the compromised airway and potential immediate feeding difficulties.
- Micrognathia is generally seen in one of two settings: either as an isolated disorder or as part of a craniofacial syndrome. It is also seen in aneuploid fetuses.
- During fetal life, if the mandible remains hypoplastic, the position of the developing tongue against the base of the cranium will prevent fusion of the medially growing palatal shelves and therefore result in a cleft palate.
- The diagnosis of micrognathia is often subjective unless there is marked mandibular hypoplasia. Sagittal views of the fetal face are best to assess the facial profile to make the diagnosis.
- Micrognathia is associated with many conditions. It is frequently associated with other fetal abnormalities and features in particular genetic syndromes. The liquor volume may also be increased, reflecting impaired fetal swallowing.
- Karyotyping should be offered. Termination of pregnancy may be an option particularly if the micrognathia is severe or if additional anomalies are present.
- Delivery should take place in a tertiary setting or where expertise for neonatal intubation is available. The mode of delivery would depend on standard obstetric considerations.
- The long-term outcome depends on the underlying diagnosis or on the presence of additional anomalies. Orthodontic and maxillofacial surgery is often required for severe cases.
- The risk of recurrence depends on whether or not the micrognathia is associated with a particular genetic syndrome.

Cystic hygroma/lymphangioma
- Cystic hygroma is a rare congenital malformation of the lymphatic system (Fig. 13.3) and has an incidence of between 1 in 6000 and 1 in 16 000 births. Among aborted fetuses, the incidence may be as high as 1 in 300.
- Cystic hygromas are thought to develop because of the failure of the jugular lymph sacs to join the lymphatic system. Both sexes are equally affected.
- The literature suggests that 50%–65% are usually present at birth and 80%–90% are diagnosed by the end of the second year of life. Approximately 75% occur in the neck, usually in the posterior triangle, more commonly on the left side. 20% occur in the axillary region.
- Chromosome abnormalities are present in almost 70% of cases with Turner syndrome and Down syndrome particularly common. There is also an association with non-chromosomal conditions (Noonan syndrome, multiple pterygium syndrome).
- Once detected, a careful search for additional abnormalities is vital. Karyotyping should always be offered. The presence of hydrops is a poor prognostic feature with a perinatal mortality rate >80%. Fetal echocardiography should be performed.

13

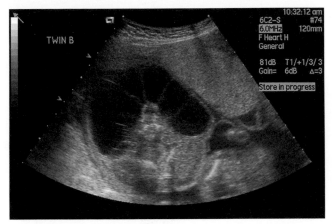

Fig. 13.3. Large cystic hygroma with septae.

- Termination of pregnancy is an option, particularly if hydrops is present or if the fetus is aneuploid. Referral to a geneticist may be appropriate in selected cases.
- The parents should be counseled by a pediatric surgeon and fully appraised of the risks of surgery.
- There is an increased incidence of preterm labor and polyhydramnios, particularly if the cystic hygroma impairs fetal swallowing. In very large lesions, obstruction of the pharynx and larynx may occur making intubation very difficult. The EXIT procedure (*Ex-utero Intrapartum Treatment*) may be required.
- Surgery is usually considered as the optimal mode of treatment. Dissection can be difficult and tedious because of the possible involvement of surrounding vital structures. Complete excision is not possible in approximately 60% of cases.
- Some cases may be suitable for intrauterine sclerotherapy using OK-432, although there is very little data on the long-term effects on the fetus.
- The long-term outcome depends on the presence of any other abnormalities and/or the ability to achieve complete excision of the cystic hygroma.

Fetal goiter
- Fetal goiter is a diffuse enlargement of the thyroid gland, which can occur in hyperthyroid, hypothyroid, or even in euthyroid states.
- Fetal thyroid dysfunction is related to passage across the placental barrier of TSH–receptor antibodies or anti-thyroid medication. The fetal thyroid only becomes responsive to exogenous stimulation

HEAD AND NECK ABNORMALITIES

(maternal thyroid antibody) in the second trimester. Goiters are therefore unlikely to be detected prior to 22 weeks' gestation.

- To assess fetal thyroid function, fetal ultrasound at 28–32 weeks should be performed if there is evidence of active maternal Graves' disease (elevated maternal thyroid antibody levels, or increased maternal requirement for anti-thyroid medication).

- Without treatment, fetal hyperthyroidism can result in 50% perinatal mortality.

- The typical ultrasound features of a goiter include a symmetric sometimes lobulated mass in the anterior neck. The fetal neck may sometimes be persistently hyperextended. Polyhydramnios may be present if the goiter is large enough to impair swallowing.

- Differential diagnoses include thyroid gland cyst, cystic hygroma, enlarged thymus, cervical meningocele, or cervical neuroblastoma.

- Features of fetal hyper- or hypothyroidism should be looked for. Some signs of hyperthyroidism include tachycardia, hydrops, or fetal growth restriction. Hypothyroid fetuses may have cardiomegaly, heart block, or even hydrops. These features are usually not specific enough to make an accurate assessment of the fetal thyroid status.

- Fetal blood sampling may be required to establish the fetal thyroid status. Direct fetal treatment with either anti-thyroid medication or with thyroxine may be necessary.

- An enlarged goiter causing persistent neck extension may sometimes preclude a vaginal delivery and Caesarean section may be required. There may be a significant upper airway obstruction of the baby at birth and the EXIT procedure may occasionally be required.

- Most cases of hyperthyroid goiter resolve within 3 months as the thyroid stimulating antibodies are cleared.

CARDIOVASCULAR ABNORMALITIES

Cardiovascular system

- The fetal heart develops from the splanchnic mesoderm and, in its earliest and most rudimentary form, is represented by two tubes, which subsequently fuse and then canalize. Repeated rotations and septations then occur which ultimately results in a four-chamber organ. The myocardium increases by cell division until birth and subsequent growth is due to cell hypertrophy.
- A fetal heart beat can be detected by 22 days and, by 8 weeks' gestation, some degree of neurogenic regulation occurs as a result of innnervation by the sympathetic and parasympathetic nervous systems. However, the fetal myocardium, in general, shows immaturity of structure, function, and sympathetic innervation relative to the adult heart.
- The fetal heart has a limited capacity to increase its output, as it normally operates at the top of its cardiac function curve (the Frank–Starling mechanism does operate in the fetal heart). An increase in fetal heart rate can increase the cardiac output albeit modestly, but bradycardia can significantly compromise its function.
- Congenital heart disease affects 6–8 per 1000 live births, at least half of which should be detectable before birth.

Distribution and pattern of the fetal circulation

- Much of the data on distribution and volume of fetal blood flow comes from animal studies. In the fetus, the right and left ventricles pump blood into the arterial circulation in parallel. The characteristic anatomical feature of the fetal circulation in contrast to the adult, is the presence of several vascular shunts (foramen ovale, ductus venosus, and ductus arteriosus), which ensure that most of the blood bypasses the fetal lungs and is shunted towards the the placenta (Fig. 14.1).
- The blood volume in the human fetus is approximately 10%–12% of body weight compared with 7%–8% in the adult. The main reason for this is the large reservoir of blood within the placenta. The fetoplacental blood volume in human fetuses is 110–115 ml/kg and the estimated volume in the fetal body is approximately 80 ml/kg.
- The systemic systolic pressure in human fetuses increases from 15–20 mmHg at 16 weeks to 30–40 mmHg at 28 weeks. A similar increase is also seen for diastolic pressure which is <5 mmHg at 16–18 weeks and 5–15 mmHg at 19–26 weeks. Umbilical venous pressures, in contrast, change only slightly (4.5 mmHg at 18 weeks to 6 mmHg at term).
- Approximately 40% (200 ml/kg per min) of fetal cardiac output is distributed to the placental circulation and a similar volume will return to the heart via the umbilical venous system.

14

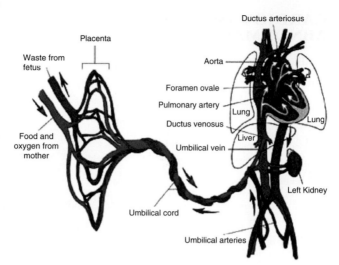

Fig. 14.1. Fetal circulation.

- After entering the intra-abdominal portion of the umbilical vein, a portion of umbilical venous flow supplies the liver, but the rest passes through the ductus venosus and into the heart. The ductus venosus is a slender trumpet-like shunt that connects the intrahepatic portion of the umbilical vein to the inferior vena cava at its inlet into the heart. Changes in the umbilical venous pressure causes the blood to accelerate from a mean of 10–22 cm/s in the umbilical vein to 60–65 cm/s as it enters the ductus venosus and flows towards the inferior vena cava and the heart.
- There is preferential streaming of blood from the ductus venosus in a dorsal and leftward direction in the inferior vena cava so that blood flows through the foramen ovale and left atrium, then through the left ventricle and aorta. This more highly oxygenated blood (SaO_2 60%), therefore, perfuses the coronary arteries and the head and neck vessels. Despite preferential streaming of blood in the inferior vena cava and through the foramen ovale, there is still some mixing of blood in the right atrium which passes into the right ventricle. However, the blood in the left atrium (SaO_2 70%) is still of significantly higher saturation compared with the right atrium (SaO_2 20%).
- Blood returning to the heart, from the inferior and superior vena cava and coronary sinus, flows preferentially through the right atrium and into the right ventricle. This blood then enters the pulmonary artery and is diverted through the ductus arteriosus into the descending aorta. Almost 40% of the cardiac output is directed though this

shunt. The lungs receive approximately 13% of cardiac output at mid-gestation and 20%–25% after 30 weeks.

14

- Patency of the ductus arteriosus is regulated by both dilatory and constrictive factors and by the impedance of the pulmonary vascular bed, which is under the control of prostaglandin I_2. There is a degree of basal tonic constriction that is augmented by endothelin. Circulating prostaglandins, particularly prostaglandin E_2, is crucial in maintaining patency, and nitric oxide also has a dilatory effect prior to the third trimester.
- Sensitivity to prostaglandins antagonists is highest in the third trimester and is enhanced by glucocorticoids and fetal stress. The ductus arteriosus closes within 2 days of birth. The main trigger for its closure is the increase in arterial oxygen concentrations, which rise when the fetus makes the transition to extrauterine life and regular respiration is established.
- Severe atrioventricular valve or semilunar valve regurgitation in utero may affect the filling of the contralateral ventricle. Impairment of forward flow at any level (atrial, ventricular, or arterial) will lead to shunting of blood to the opposite side via the foramen ovale (and a ventricular septal defect, if present). Markedly reduced right ventricular output will cause a reversal of flow in the ductus arteriosus to direct the blood from the aorta towards the pulmonary circulation.
- If left ventricular output is severely compromised, flow in the aortic arch is reversed and the blood from the ductus arteriosus is directed towards the head and neck vessels, and the coronary arteries.
- Impaired right atrial and ventricular filling leads to altered Doppler waveform patterns in the systemic veins, particularly if the foramen ovale is restrictive. Reduced oxygen content of the blood supplying the fetal brain due to lesions such as transposition of great arteries, hypoplastic left heart syndrome, may increase cerebral blood flow as a result of vasodilatation.

Changes at birth
- In the human newborn, the ductus venosus is functionally closed within a few hours although it takes almost 3 weeks to permanently obliterate. This may take longer in preterm infants or in cases of persistent pulmonary hypertension or cardiac malformations. The foramen ovale is also functionally closed shortly after birth, but permanent closure is a slow process and normally does not occur for up to 12 months.
- Within minutes after the onset of respiration, pulmonary vascular resistance decreases and pulmonary blood flow increases tenfold. Right ventricular output is therefore directed more to the lungs, and the right and left sides of the heart begin to pump in series converting to a more adult pattern of circulation.
- High cardiac output after birth is required principally to sustain global body perfusion and to support the increase in metabolism required to maintain thermoregulation.

14

Fetal echocardiography

- Congenital heart abnormalities are the commonest fetal malformations and have a familial association. Cardiac malformations are also associated with a wide variety of fetal and maternal conditions and medications.
- Fetal echocardiography should be considered for the following: first-degree relative with congenital heart disease (1 previous sibling affected 2%–4% risk, 10% if ≥2 previous siblings affected, 5%–12% if mother and 1%–3% if father affected), maternal insulin-dependent diabetes (3%–4%), autoimmune antibodies (anti-Ro and anti-La), drug therapy (lithium 10%) or epilepsy (4%–7% risk with monotherapy, 15% risk with polytherapy), monochorionic twins (4% risk), increased NT ≥3.5 mm (3% rising to 23% if >5.5 mm) and high-risk structural anomalies (tracheo-esophageal fistula (15%–40% risk), duodenal atresia (17% risk), omphalocele (20%–30% risk), and diaphragmatic hernia (10%–20% risk).
- Examination should include confirmation of situs, four-chamber view, great arterial crossover, three-vessel view of the transverse aortic, ductal arches, and superior vena cava.
- Detection of any cardiac abnormality should prompt detailed evaluation for extracardiac anomalies. Karyotyping should be offered (risk 1%–50% depending on lesion. Concomitant 22q deletion testing by FISH should be performed for outflow tract abnormalities (risk 1% risk overall, but 10% with outflow tract lesions).
- Counseling should be multidisciplinary (fetal medicine specialist, pediatric cardiologist, and cardiothoracic surgeon). For major abnormalities, or if associated with other structural anomalies, or if aneuploid, termination of pregnancy should be offered.
- Follow-up echocardiography and obstetric scans essential to monitor progression, fetal growth and well-being. Most cases will require delivery at a tertiary center. For most abnormalities, mode of delivery may be decided on standard obstetric grounds.

Aortic stenosis

- Aortic stenosis accounts for 4%–6% of all cardiovascular abnormalities and is four times more common in males. It has an incidence of 3–4 per 10 000 live births.
- Aortic stenosis may be either subvalvular, valvular, or supravalvular. Stenosis secondary to valve abnormalities are usually due to cusp malformations seen in unicuspid or bicuspid aortic valves. The incidence of bicuspid aortic valves is approximately 1 in 100 newborns.
- Obstruction of the left ventricular outflow tract increases pressure load to the left ventricle and volume load to the right ventricle. Critical aortic stenosis causes reduced left ventricular output and increased diastolic filling pressure, which then causes hypertrophy followed by dilatation of the left ventricle.
- In the absence of mitral valve regurgitation, blood flow through the foramen ovale is then reversed (left to right shunting). The raised

left ventricular diastolic pressure may compromise coronary blood flow and lead to myocardial fibrosis. Ultimately, left ventricular hypoplasia develops and the right ventricle takes over to support the pulmonary, placental, and systemic circulations. Fetuses with restrictive foramen do not do well, due to the lack of adequate left-to-right shunting at the atrial level. Resulting left atrial hypertension can alter pulmonary venous return and cause pulmonary vascular hypertension.

- Although left ventricular growth may be facilitated by the presence of mitral valve regurgitation due to increased preload, fetuses seem to tolerate such lesions less well possibly due to its effect on the filling of the right ventricle.

- Critical aortic stenosis can cause coronary hypoperfusion, subendocardial ischemia, and significant metabolic acidosis. The development of hydrops fetalis carries a very poor prognosis.

- Differential diagnoses include hypoplastic left heart syndrome, co-arctation of the aorta, and cardiomyopathy. Hypoplastic left heart syndrome is frequently associated with both aortic and mitral valve atresia.

- The procedure of choice for critical aortic stenosis for candidates thought suitable for a biventricular repair is neonatal balloon valvuloplasty. Currently published outcomes for treatment in the first week of life vary widely, with reports ranging from 56% mortality with 44% of survivors requiring re-intervention. Ten-year survival rates are less than 50%.

- Fetal valvuloplasty has been used with varying degrees of success. The rationale for in utero therapy includes the belief that restoration of flow across the valve improves growth of the left ventricle, secondary damage is therefore limited, and finally that a biventricular circulation provides a better quality of life than a univentricular one.

- Fetal intervention has been shown to restore forward flow through the aortic arch in cases of critical aortic stenosis and may improve the delivery of blood flow to the cerebral circulation. This may theoretically reduce the risk of neurologic damage associated with major cardiac defects, but the evidence for this is still lacking.

- Fetal aortic valvuloplasty, when technically successful, improves left ventricular systolic function and left heart Doppler characteristics. Furthermore, initial results suggest that prenatal decompression of the left atrium may be associated with greater early hospital survival. Long-term outcome data is still lacking.

- In many congenital heart centers, transcatheter balloon valvuloplasty is the initial procedure of choice in newborns with congenital aortic stenosis that are either duct dependent or have low cardiac output. Other surgical options that may become necessary include open valvuloplasty, Ross–Konno procedure, or the Norwood procedure (if a univentricular repair is required).

- Postdelivery patency of the ductus arteriosus should be maintained with prostaglandin E2 and any associated metabolic acidosis corrected. An early neonatal echo should be performed to confirm the cardiac abnormality and treatment then planned.

14

Pulmonary stenosis

- This is a fairly common abnormality with varying presentations. Often, the diagnosis is made well after delivery. It has an incidence of approximately 1 in 1500 live births.
- Pulmonary stenosis may be isolated, occur in association with other abnormalities (Fallot's tetralogy), occur in association with genetic syndromes (Williams' syndrome, Noonan syndrome) or secondary to congenital rubella infection.
- Narrowing of the pulmonary valve can lead to hypertrophy of the right ventricle and, in severe cases, cause hypoplasia of the right ventricle.
- Ultrasound features include a smaller right ventricle, right atrial enlargement, valve thickening, poststenotic dilatation, and reversed flow across the ductal arch. Frequently, detection of these abnormalities is extremely difficult and the diagnosis is only made after birth.
- Pulmonary stenosis may progress in utero, resulting in tricuspid regurgitation, heart failure and hydrops.
- Once the abnormality is suspected, serial scans are necessary to assess progression. Karyotyping should be offered. Counseling by a fetal/pediatric cardiologist should be arranged. Termination of pregnancy should be discussed in cases of critical stenosis, hypoplastic right heart, or if hydrops is present.
- Fetal intervention has recently been offered to prevent or slow the progression of ventricular hypoplasia during the second and third trimester and to optimize right (and left) ventricular function, particularly where there is severe tricuspid regurgitation and abnormalities of the fetal circulation, including hydrops.
- It is difficult to be certain about the efficacy of in utero intervention and each case needs to be considered on an individual basis. There is a high procedure-related loss rate and referral to a fetal medicine unit, and discussion with a fetal medicine specialist and interventional pediatric cardiologist is essential before proceeding with this option.
- Delivery of the baby should take place in a tertiary unit. The ductus arteriosus should be kept patent with a prostaglandin E_2 infusion. Early echocardiography to confirm the diagnosis and to exclude other cardiac malformations should be performed.
- Cardiac catheterization and balloon valvoplasty are the treatment of choice, although some cases may require open heart surgery.

Hypoplastic left heart syndrome (HLHS)

- HLHS is a major congenital heart anomaly accounting for 1% of congenital cardiac abnormalities. However, it is responsible for 25% of all cardiac deaths in the first week of life. Without treatment, newborn babies with hypoplastic left heart syndrome (HLHS) usually die within the first week of life.
- HLHS is the end result of a spectrum of conditions, which include aortic valve stenosis/atresia, mitral valve stenosis/atresia, proximal aortic hypoplasia and left ventricular hypoplasia (Figs. 14.2 and 14.3).
- The entire systemic circulation is supplied by the right ventricle. The majority of the cardiac output goes through the pulmonary artery,

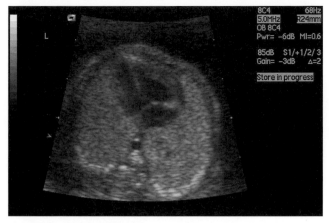

Fig. 14.2. Hypoplastic left heart.

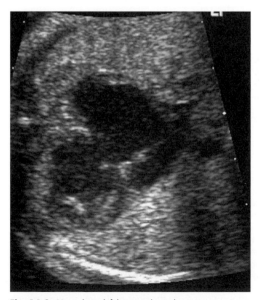

Fig. 14.3. Hypoplastic left heart and mitral atresia.

ductus arteriosus, and enters the aorta. However, after birth, when pulmonary vascular resistance falls and the ductus arteriosus closes, the neonate develops profound systemic hypoperfusion/hypotension and acidosis.

- Important associated anomalies include pulmonary venous return abnormalities. Central nervous system anomalies including agenesis of the corpus callosum, microcephaly, and holoprosencephaly have been reported.

- Some HLHS variants are not easily recognizable at first and become apparent only on postnatal evaluation or at follow-up. If the diagnosis is missed prenatally, infants generally are born at term, and initially appear healthy. With closure of the arterial duct, systemic perfusion becomes decreased, resulting in hypoxemia, acidosis, and shock.

- If a diagnosis of aortic stenosis is made, the fetus should be monitored carefully for the development of HLHS. Assessment of the interatrial septum (IAS) should be made to detect any impairment in left-to-right flow.

- HLHS is associated with aneuploidy, genetic syndromes (Holt–Oram, Noonan syndrome, etc.), and extracardiac abnormalities.

- The patient should be referred to a tertiary center and jointly managed by a fetal medicine specialist and pediatric cardiologist. Karyotyping is indicated. Termination of pregnancy should be discussed with parents, as the outcome for the majority of cases is very poor.

- Following birth, the baby requires prostaglandin E2 to maintain patency of the ductus arteriosus and oxygen supplementation used judiciously, so as to avoid significant reduction in pulmonary vascular pressure. The diagnosis should be confirmed with a neonatal echo and the baby reviewed by a cardiothoracic surgeon regarding timing of surgery. Ionotropic agents and correction of acidosis may be required.

- Currently, there are two treatment options: primary cardiac trans-plantation or a series of staged functionally univentricular palliations (Norwood procedure). The treatment chosen is dependent on the preference of the institution and its experience. Although survival following initial surgical intervention has improved significantly over the last 20 years, there is still significant mortality and morbidity.

- The first stage of palliation, or the Norwood operation, is performed at birth. The second stage is a bidirectional Glenn operation, usually undertaken at 6 to 8 months of age. The third, and final, stage is the Fontan operation, which can be performed between the ages of 18 months and 4 years. The highest risk of mortality is following the initial operation with some series quoting a 30% death rate.

Hypoplastic right heart syndrome
- This anomaly is due to pulmonary valve atresia with an intact interventricular septum (PA-IVS). Occasionally, the tricuspid valve is also atretic. Blood flows from the right to the left atrium through the foramen ovale and then into the left ventricle and aorta. The left

ventricle supplies both the systemic as well as the pulmonary circulation (by retrograde flow through the ductus arteriosus).

- Fistulas between the coronary arteries and the right ventricle decompress the right ventricle by carrying desaturated systemic venous blood back to the aorta. They can also supply the coronary arteries and, in some cases, may be the sole source of coronary blood flow.

- The malformation is suspected if there is obvious discrepancy in size between the two ventricles. The diagnosis may not be clear at the initial investigation, and serial scans may be required to detect evolution of the condition.

- Fetuses having pulmonary atresia with intact ventricular septum show right heart hypoplasia with an overall 5-year survival of only 65% in a large population-based series. There is significant morbidity, and postnatal biventricular circulation can be achieved in only 32%–55%.

- If the diagnosis is suspected, referral to a tertiary center and review by a pediatric cardiologist is essential. Karyotyping may be indicated if additional anomalies are present. The overall risk for aneuploidy is low. Termination of pregnancy should be discussed. The presence of hydrops worsens the prognosis.

- If the right ventricular hypoplasia is due to progressive pulmonary stenosis, consideration may be given for in utero pulmonary valvuloplasty. There is limited experience with fetal therapy for pulmonary valve stenosis compared with aortic valve disease. Technical success rates are high in some groups, but initial results suggest that the outcomes of these small series seem similar to the natural history of the condition. This is often due to growth failure of the tricuspid valve. Anecdotally, however, there is dramatic improvement in the circulation of some fetuses, with resolution of hydrops.

Atrioventricular septal defect (AVSD)

- AVSDs covers a spectrum of congenital heart malformations characterized by a common atrioventricular junction coexisting with deficient atrioventricular septation. In ostium primum atrial septal defect (ASD) there are separate atrioventricular valvular orifices despite a common junction, while in complete AVSD there is a common valve (Fig. 14.4).

- The incidence ranges from 21–34 per 10 000 live births. There is a strong association (30%–50%) with Down syndrome. Additional cardiac malformations are present in more than 70% of cases.

- Three different genetic patterns are described in AVSD: the association with Down syndrome, as an autosomal dominant trait, and isolated. Cases of autosomal dominant inheritance are not linked to chromosome 21.

- Associated cardiac anomalies include subaortic stenosis, ventricular hypoplasia, tetralogy of Fallot, atrial isomerism, double outlet right ventricle, pulmonary stenosis, etc. AVSD is present in almost 17% of cases of tetralogy of Fallot. Up to 45% of cases diagnosed in utero are associated with the heterotaxy syndrome and will have left atrial

14

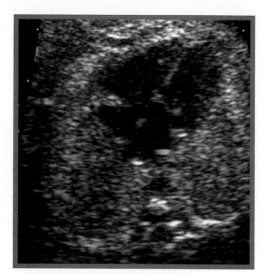

Fig. 14.4. Atrioventricular septal defect.

isomerism. In left atrial isomerism associated with an AVSD, complete heart block is common.

- The combination of left atrial isomerism, AVSD, and complete heart block with hydrops, has a very poor perinatal prognosis.
- The key diagnostic feature on the four-chamber view of the heart is the presence of a common atrioventricular valve.
- Once the abnormality is detected, referral to a tertiary center and paediatric cardiologist is advisable. Karyotyping is essential and careful assessment of the fetus for additional anomalies is important. Termination of pregnancy should be offered for large lesions with fetal hydrops, if aneuploidy is detected or if there are other major associated anomalies.
- Patients that elect to continue with the pregnancy should be referred to a pediatric cardiac surgeon for further counseling.
- Mode and timing of delivery is on standard obstetric grounds.
- There is no fetal intervention for this anomaly. The mainstay of treatment is surgical correction of the defect. The objectives of surgical correction are to close all septal defects and to repair the atrioventricular valve. Surgical correction in complete AVSD should be performed within the first few months of life and certainly before 6 months in order to avoid the development of pulmonary vascular disease. Operative mortality is low (<5%). The overall 10-year survival is >80%.

Fetal arrhythmias

- Rhythm abnormalities occur in 2% of fetuses, the vast majority being isolated atrial or ventricular premature contractions.
- The majority of fetal tachycardias are supraventricular in origin, of which supraventricular tachycardia (SVT) associated with an AV accessory pathway is most common.
- Fetal SVT due to an accessory AV pathway is associated with ventricular rates typically of 230–280 bpm. At birth, 10% of affected fetuses have Wolff–Parkinson–White syndrome.
- Atrial flutter is usually identified late in gestation with atrial rates ranging from 300–550 bpm with variable AV conduction and thus ventricular rates. The very high atrial rates and slower ventricular rates are usually confirmed through M mode tracings or systemic venous Doppler demonstration of the atrial wave rates.
- Hydrops fetalis is present or develops in 40%–50% of fetuses with SVT. SVT results in reduced diastolic filling time, which leads to increasing atrial and central venous pressures.
- Treatment is mainly reserved for fetuses with heart failure or for those in whom the risk of developing heart failure is high. Fetuses at highest risk of developing heart failure are those with more persistent SVT, those with earlier onset of SVT (<32 weeks), and those with structural heart disease (which complicates 10% of supraventricular tachyarrhythmias).
- Most fetal SVTs can be treated successfully through maternal/transplacental administration of antiarrhythmia medications. Many different drugs can be used, including digoxin, propranolol, flecainide, sotalol, verapamil, and amiodarone. Digoxin alone has been associated with an 80%–85% success rate in the treatment of fetal SVT and 60%–65% in the treatment of atrial flutter in the absence of fetal heart failure.
- Cardioversion to sinus rhythm can take several days, sometimes much longer, particularly if the fetus is hydropic with placentomegaly.
- Occasionally, direct fetal treatment with fetal blood sampling and injection of antiarrhythmic medication may be required for refractory SVT despite adequate and prolonged maternal treatment.
- Postdelivery the baby will require an electrocardiogram (ECG) and echo and continuation of antiarrhythmic treatment. Occasionally, cardiac pacing may be necessary.
- Fetal bradycardia is usually diagnosed when the ventricular rate is <110 bpm. The most common cause of fetal bradycardia is sinus bradycardia. Rarely, it may be a sign of long QT syndrome.
- Fetal AV block is another cause of fetal bradycardia. Usually, it presents with complete AV block but occasionally second-degree and, more rarely first-degree AV block.
- Fetal AV block is associated with maternal autoantibodies in approximately 40% of cases, structural heart disease in 45%–48% of cases, and is isolated and of unclear etiology in 4%–10% of cases.
- Transplacental passage of maternal autoantibodies (anti-SSA/Ro and/or anti-SSB/La) is believed to cause inflammation and fibrosis to the conducting system and endocardium. Although these

14

CARDIOVASCULAR ABNORMALITIES

14

antibodies are found in women with clinical autoimmune disease, including Sjögren syndrome and SLE, 70%–80% of the mothers of affected fetuses have no clinical autoimmune disease at the time of fetal diagnosis.

- The risk of complete heart block in an anti-Ro positive mother is 2%–5%. 90% of mothers of affected children have anti-Ro antibodies and 50%–70% are positive for anti-La antibodies.
- Between 15% and 20% of fetuses with auto-immune mediated AV block have additional more diffuse myocardial disease, which can lead to endocardial fibrosis and ventricular dysfunction. A ventricular rate of <50 bpm is associated with increased mortality.
- Maternal treatments with dexamathasone, plasmapheresis, beta sympathomimetics, and immunoglobulin have all been used with varying degrees of success.

Tetralogy of Fallot
- Tetralogy of Fallot (ToF) occurs in approximately 1 in 3600 live births and accounts for 3.5% of infants born with congenital heart disease.
- It comprises a VSD, right ventricular outflow tract obstruction, the aorta overriding the interventricular septum, and right ventricular hypertrophy (Fig. 14.5).
- The spectrum of severity is wide ranging from right outflow tract obstruction to pulmonary atresia. The VSD is usually perimembranous and is large and non-restrictive. Other VSDs may occasionally be present (muscular inlet defects or a complete AVSD usually seen in Down syndrome). Other variants include absent pulmonary valve syndrome and pulmonary atresia with multiple aorto-pulmonary collaterals (MAPCAs).
- Fetal diagnosis is made when a large VSD with aortic override, a smaller diameter of the pulmonary outflow tract, and a relatively larger aorta are seen. Hypertrophy of the right ventricle is not a prenatal feature, unlike in childhood.
- The size of the main pulmonary artery and its ratio to the ascending aorta in mid trimester reflects the severity of the right outflow tract obstruction.
- Growth of the pulmonary vessels throughout pregnancy may be normal or reduced. The ductus arteriosus is smaller than normal in fetuses with ToF, but forward (right to left) flow is usually maintained. The presence of left to right ductal flow indicates severe outflow tract obstruction or pulmonary atresia.
- Absent pulmonary valves are seen in 3%–6% of cases. 15% of cases may be associated with the DiGeorge syndrome caused by a deletion on the long arm of chromosome 22 (22q11.2).
- Once the diagnosis is suspected, referral to a pediatric cardiologist is essential. Karyotyping should be offered (including 22q deletion studies). Additional anomalies should be excluded. Serial scans to document fetal pulmonary artery growth and ductal flow patterns are

14

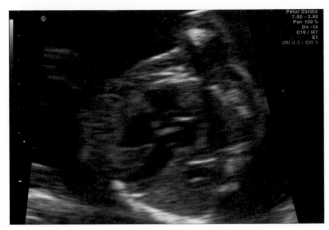

Fig. 14.5. Tetralogy of Fallot with overiding aorta and ventricular septal defect.

essential for counseling and planning appropriate management of the newborn baby.

- Termination of pregnancy should be discussed if the diagnosis is made early. The development of hydrops is a poor prognostic sign. Delivery should occur in a tertiary unit.
- The severity of the right outflow tract obstruction determines the clinical presentation. If severe, a duct-dependent pulmonary circulation is present, and a prostaglandin E_2 infusion may be required to maintain ductal patency.
- Surgical repair is through a transatrial, transpulmonary approach whenever possible. There is no benefit in delaying elective repair of ToF after the end of the first year. The 5-year survival rate is almost 95%. However, sudden death can occur in 6% of patients long term.

Transposition of the great arteries (TGA)

- In this abnormality the aorta arises from the morphological right ventricle (RV), and the pulmonary artery arises from the morphological left ventricle (LV). The aorta tends to be on the right and anterior, and the great arteries are parallel rather than crossing as they do in the normal heart. This is also known as d-TGA.
- In corrected TGA or l-TGA the right atrium is connected to the left ventricle and then to the pulmonary artery, and the left atrium is connected to the right ventricle and blood then flows to the aorta.

14

- Communication between the parallel systemic and pulmonary circulations (atrial septal defect, a ventricular septal defect (VSD), or at the great arterial level (patent ductus arteriosus)), is necessary to ensure that systemic blood enters the pulmonary circulation for oxygenation and to allow oxygenated blood from the pulmonary circuit to enter the systemic circulation.
- The most common associated lesion is a VSD, which occurs in 50% of cases and is usually associated with subvalvular pulmonary stenosis.
- It is one of the most common causes of neonatal cyanosis. If the ventricular septum is intact, the baby is usually cyanotic on day 1 of life. If circulatory mixing occurs via a patent ductus arteriosus, physiological closure of the ductus causes abrupt cyanosis and clinical deterioration.
- The diagnosis is made on examination of the fetal cardiac outflow tracts. Failure to visualize the normal crossover of vessels and/or the presence of parallel large vessels should lead to suspicion of the diagnosis. Differentiation between corrected and uncorrected TGA is extremely difficult prenatally. Careful examination of the right and left ventricles may aid in the diagnosis.
- Most fetuses tolerate this abnormality well in utero. The presence of additional cardiac abnormalities (pulmonary stenosis, VSD) may cause cardiac failure and hydrops and worsen the prognosis.
- Once the diagnosis is suspected, the patient should be referred to a pediatric cardiologist for further assessment. Karyotyping and 22q deletion studies should be performed. Termination of pregnancy should be discussed if the diagnosis is made early or if there are additional anomalies present.
- Delivery must take place in a tertiary center. The mode of delivery is on standard obstetric grounds. Early postdelivery echocardiography should be performed to confirm the diagnosis.
- Postdelivery, most babies will deteriorate and become cyanosed and a prostaglandin E_2 infusion may be required to maintain ductal patency. If an intact ventricular septum is present and there is inadequate mixing of blood at an atrial level, an emergency percutaneous Rashkind atrial balloon septostomy may be required. This creates a bigger atrial septal defect, which can improve oxygenation until definitive surgery can be performed.
- Surgery is indicated for all babies and is best done early in the neonatal period. The arterial switch procedure involves dividing the pulmonary artery and re-anastomosis to the right ventricular outflow tract and dividing the aorta with re-anastomosis to the left ventricular outflow tract. The operative mortality is <10%. 5-year survival is approximately 85%.

MONOCHORIONIC TWINS

- Monozygous twins arise from one fertilized egg in contrast to dizygous twins that arise from two separately fertilized eggs.
- Monozygotic twins occur spontaneously in about 1 in 250 births and increase with ovulation induction techniques. They also increase in proportion to the number of blastocysts transferred during in vitro fertilization.
- Dizygotic twinning appears to be influenced by race, genetic factors, maternal age, fertility-enhancing drugs, folic acid supplementation, and maternal nutritional status.
- If cellular division occurs in the first 3 days after fertilization, the monozygous twins may be dichorionic diamniotic (25%–30%), between 4 and 7 days, monochorionic diamniotic (70%–75%) and between 7–14 days, monochorionic monoamniotic (1%–2%).
- Dizygotic twins have separate placentae and membranes (dichorionic diamniotic), although these may be fused and occasionally even have vascular connections.
- Conjoined twins are always monozygotic. They result from incomplete monozygotic twinning and have an incidence of 1 in 100 000 births or 1 in 400 monozygotic twin births. There is an excess of females among conjoined twins. They are classified by site of attachment.
- Conjoined twins are thought to develop after 14 days of embryonic development. 50% of conjoined twins have major structural anomalies with a high risk of intrauterine, neonatal, and infant death. Miscarriage and preterm labor are also more common.
- The causes of monozygotic twinning in human beings are unknown, athough there is an increased incidence following artificial reproductive techniques.
- In monozygotic twins, congenital anomalies (particularly cardiac malformations) occur more frequently (3.9%). 10% of monozygotic twins are born with a congenital malformation.
- Single intrauterine fetal demise in a monochorionic pregnancy may be associated with >20% risk for multicystic encephalomalacia in the surviving cotwin.

Pregnancy complications in monozygous twins

Twin–twin transfusion syndrome (TTTS)

- TTTS occurs in approximately 15% of all monochorionic pregnancies, and results from intertwin transfusion across shared placental vascular anastomoses. Untreated, it is associated with a perinatal mortality rate of over 90%. Long-term neurologic and cardiovascular dysfunction are potential sequelae of untreated or aggressive disease.
- TTTS is due to unbalanced deep arteriovenous anastomoses without compensatory superficial anastomoses. Three types of anastomoses have been described – Arterial–arterial (AA), Vein–vein (VV) and Arterial–venous (AV) (Figs. 15.1 and 15.2).

15

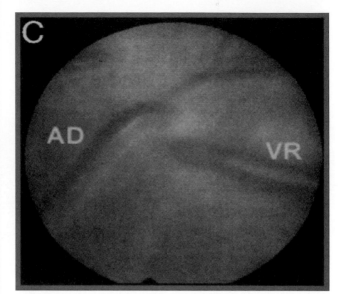

Fig. 15.1. Artery-to-vein anastomosis. See color plate section.

- AA and VV are bidirectional superficial anastomoses that run on the surface of the placenta. AV are deep anastomoses, where a closely related unpaired artery and vein pierce the chorionic plate to supply a shared placental cotyledon.
- Transfusion through the unidirectional AV anastomoses creates hydrostatic differences between the twins. The donor responds with oliguria, and the recipient responds with polyuria and polyhydramnios. The increase in the recipient's blood volume and atrial distension results in increased secretion of atrial natriuretic peptide (ANP) and vasopressin. Hypovolemia, renal underperfusion, and oliguria in the donor may lead to renal changes (diffuse renal tubular atrophy progressing to renal tubular dysgenesis) causing renal failure at birth in a small proportion of donors.
- Maternal hyperaldosteronism is exaggerated in women with TTTS, maintaining plasma volume due to increasing third space loss.
- Urine production in the donor finally ceases resulting in a "stuck twin" (Figs. 15.3 and 15.4). Vasoconstrictor peptides, such as the renin–angiotensin system (RAS) mediators increase significantly, resulting in elevated vascular resistance in the donor's placental territory aggravating the growth impairment. Similar cord levels of renin and aldosterone are seen in the recipient (despite discordant renal expression of renin between the two fetuses) because of transfer

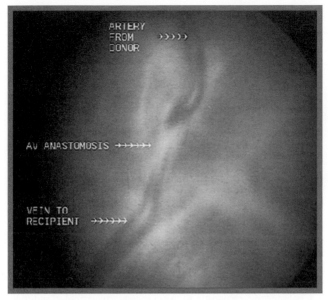

Fig. 15.2. Artery to vein anastomosis on chorionic plate. See color plate section.

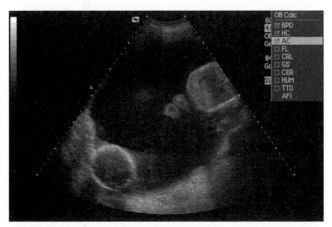

Fig. 15.3. Oligohydramnios–polyhydramnios sequence in twin-to-twin transfusion syndrome.

15

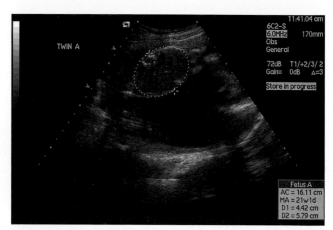

Fig. 15.4. Stuck twin (Donor).

through placental anastomosis. The increased cardiac output and systemic hypertension in the recipient worsen its cardiac function.

- Cardiomegaly secondary to biventricular hypertrophy and right ventricular systolic and biventricular diastolic dysfunction develops. Occasionally, right ventricular outflow tract obstruction may evolve (10% of recipient fetuses). If progressive, hydrops will develop. There is good evidence that the presence of an arterio-arterial anastomosis is protective against the development of TTTS (Fig. 15.5).
- Future cardiovascular function in survivors may be abnormal. Arterial compliance is reduced in surviving donors followed in childhood. Decreased arterial distensibility enhances the impedance of the affected vessels and may initiate permanent changes in the arterial structure.
- The diagnosis of TTTS is usually made on routine antenatal ultrasound when discordancy in liquor volume is detected against the background of a monochorionic pregnancy. The Quintero staging system is currently widely used both in disease classification and in planning therapy.
- In Stage I there is oligohydramnios (deepest pool <2 cm) in the donor's sac and polyhydramnios (deepest pool >8 cm) in the recipient's sac. In Stage II the donor's bladder is not visible and the donor is usually stuck.
- Doppler abnormalities (absent or reversed flow in the umbilical artery of the donor, absent "a" wave in the ductus venosus and/or pulsatile umbilical vein in the recipient) in either twin are a feature of Stage III and, when hydrops is present, it is Stage IV. In Stage V one of the twins is dead.

MONOCHORIONIC TWINS

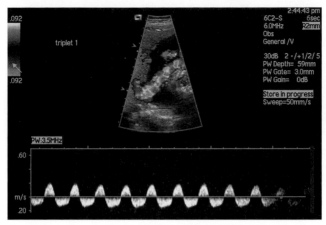

Fig. 15.5. Doppler waveform of an artery-to-artery anastomosis. See color plate section.

- Almost 70% of cases with Stage I disease will either remain stable or regress. Expectant or temporising therapy with amnioreduction may be appropriate in these cases.
- There is now, however, very good evidence that laser therapy is superior to amnioreduction or conservative management in severe TTTS (Stages III–IV) based on several observational series and randomized controlled trials.

Amnioreduction
- Amnioreduction reduces the intra-amniotic pressure and may also improve uterine perfusion and blood flow in the umbilical cord. The rationale for this technique is to prevent preterm delivery related to polyhydramnios and to improve fetal hemodynamics by decreasing pressure on the placental surface.
- Amnioreduction usually needs to be repeated weekly in up to 80% of cases because the underlying pathophysiology has not been corrected. Some (particularly early-stage disease) cases of TTTS respond well to therapeutic amnioreduction.
- The optimal management at presentation of Stage I disease is unclear. Amnioreduction may reverse the condition in as many as 20% of cases. Overall survival ranges from 38%–81% (average 60%). However, amnio reduction can lead to membrane separation, intra-amniotic bleeding and has a significant risk or membrane rupture and preterm delivery. There is an approximately 4% procedure-related risk of premature labor.

MONOCHORIONIC TWINS

15

15

- On subgroup analysis, the Eurofetus trial found that selective laser ablation was more effective as a first-line treatment of Stage I–II TTTS than was amnioreduction, with reported survivals of at least one twin of 86% in the laser group versus 58% in the amnioreduction group. However, this study contained only small numbers of Stage I disease, thereby limiting the robustness of this finding.
- It may be reasonable to use amnioreduction for stable Stage I or II disease, but the treatment of rapidly progressive early disease is still unclear. It may be better to proceed directly to fetoscopic laser treatment in these cases.
- A number of factors are possibly linked with progression of early-stage disease including early gestation at presentation, significant polyhydramnios, a small donor bladder, and absence of an artery-to-artery anastomosis.

Septostomy
- The rationale for septostomy was to equilibrate the amniotic fluid volume and thereby correct pressure differences between the two sacs.
- A multicentre randomized controlled trial comparing septostomy to amnioreduction, showed the same overall perinatal survival of 65% for both septostomy and amnioreduction.
- This procedure is no longer used for the treatment of TTTS.

Fetoscopic laser ablation of placental vascular anastomoses
- This is the treatment of choice for advanced-stage disease (stage III/IV) and has the advantage of actually dealing with the underlying mechanism (unbalanced interfetal transfusion) causing TTTS.
- The aim of laser therapy is to essentially create a functional dichorionic placenta, thereby interrupting flow between donor and recipient, and protecting either twin from hypotension in the event that one fetus dies.
- It is generally performed under local or regional anesthesia with prophylactic antibiotic cover and tocolytics.
- The first randomized controlled trial published in 2004 (Eurofetus study) to compare the safety and efficacy of laser treatment versus amnioreduction for severe TTTS diagnosed before 26 weeks showed that laser therapy resulted in higher survival rates and better neurological outcome both in the perinatal period and in the first 6 months of life. Single survivor in the laser arm was 76% versus 51% in the amnioreduction arm. Double survival was 36% for laser therapy versus 26% for amnioreduction.
- Laser therapy was beneficial across all stages, although the numbers in the early stage group were small. The rate of pregnancy loss within 7 days after the procedure was higher in the laser group than in the amnioreduction group, but not significantly so. The median gestation at delivery was 33 weeks in the laser cohort versus 29 weeks in the amnioreduction group.
- Cystic periventricular leukomalacia (PVL) occurred less frequently in the laser group (6% vs. 14%) and survival without major neurologic

15

complications at 6 months was higher in the laser group (52% vs. 32%, respectively). In cases with single intrauterine death, a favorable outcome was five times more likely in the laser group.

- Most publications now suggest perinatal survival rates after laser treatment range between 57% and 77%, with single survival between 76% and 87%. Double survival is in the region of 40%–60%. Double fetal loss is around 5%–25%. These variations probably reflect differing thresholds for offering laser treatment, operator experience, and procedure technique.

- The most frequent maternal complication following laser surgery is premature rupture of the membranes occurring in up to 28% of cases. Clinical chorioamnionitis occurs in 2% of cases, placental abruption in 2%, miscarriage following the procedure in 7%, and intra-amniotic bleeding in 8%. Amniotic fluid leakage into the maternal peritoneal cavity occurs in 2%–7% of the cases.

- Severe preterm delivery can complicate up to 29% of cases. A short cervical length (<20 mm) before treatment is an independent risk factor for preterm delivery.

- Recurrence can occur in up to 10% of the cases treated by laser (within 1 to 11 weeks). The incidence of missed anastomoses has been found to be approximately 30% on dye injection studies of placentas following laser treatment and is the most likely cause for recurrence. Close follow-up following laser treatment is therefore essential, specifically looking for evidence of recurrence, reversal, and fetal anemia.

- Recurrence may be treated by repeat laser, serial amnioreduction, selective termination, or delivery, depending on the gestation at which it occurs.

- Transient hydrops in the donor can develop very quickly in up to 25% cases. It is believed to be due to relative volume expansion following ablation of vascular anastomosis and is not associated with a poor prognosis.

- Pre-procedure umbilical artery Doppler abnormalities (absent or reversed end diastolic flow) is predictive of fetal demise of the donor. Absent or reversed end-diastolic flow in the recipient's umbilical artery is also predictive of demise if it develops following the procedure. Middle cerebral artery Doppler monitoring is necessary in survivors following surgery in order to detect anemia.

- Long-term neurodevelopmental outcome data after laser treatment is now becoming available. An overall cerebral palsy rate of 9% at 4-year follow-up has been reported. Other studies suggest that minor neurological abnormalities are present in 7% of cases with 6% having major handicap.

- The timing and mode of delivery in monochorionic pregnancies is still unclear. Many specialists recommend elective delivery between 35 and 37 weeks because of the risk of unexpected fetal death. A recent publication demonstrated that the prospective risk of unexpected antepartum stillbirth after 32 weeks was 1 in 23 in uncomplicated (structurally normal fetuses without TTTS or growth restriction) monochorionic diamniotic twin pregnancies, despite intensive fetal surveillance.

- Although vaginal delivery of monochorionic twins is not unreasonable, there is a potential risk of an acute interfetal transfusion during labor.

- There is good evidence that planned caesarean section may reduce the risk of perinatal death of twins (regardless of chorionicity) at term by approximately 75%, compared with attempting vaginal birth. This appears principally due to reducing the risk of death of the second twin due to intrapartum anoxia (3.2 per 1000).

- Given that monochorionic pregnancies are high risk in general, and the risk of unexpected fetal death is elevated in late pregnancy, there are compelling arguments for offering elective cesarean section for delivery.

- Monochorionic twins are high-risk cases and ideally should be referred for initial assessment and counseling to a tertiary fetal medicine unit. Thereafter, serial 2-weekly scans should be performed and comprehensive assessment of growth, liquor volume, and fetal Dopplers made. Immediate referral to a fetal medicine unit is important once a problem is detected.

Single fetal death in a monochorionic pregnancy
- This can result in either death (in utero or in the immediate neonatal period) in 38% of cases and intracranial lesions at birth in up to 46% of survivors.

- The mechanism of increased mortality and morbidity in the surviving cotwin is acute blood loss into the dying twin through vascular anastomoses just before, or at the time of, death when terminal hypotension occurs. Anemia in the surviving cotwin then results. Rescue transfusion of the survivor has not been shown to improve outcome.

- If intrauterine demise of one twin occurs, depending on the gestation, delivery may be an option. It is very important that the mother is counseled about the risk of neurological damage, and long-term handicap in the surviving twin, prior to delivery. This is an important medical–legal issue.

- Another approach would be to perform fetal MRI to check the surviving twin's brain, reserving the offer of termination of pregnancy if any abnormalities become evident. In general, cerebral lesions can be detected on fetal MRI approximately 3 weeks following intrauterine demise of the cotwin.

Monochorionic twins discordant for fetal anomaly
- Once an anomaly has been detected, the patient should be referred to a fetal medicine unit. The type of abnormality and any other associated malformations should be ascertained and further investigations (karyotyping, fetal echocardiography, fetal MRI) performed. If aneuploidy is confirmed, the structurally normal cotwin will be similarly affected.

- If the abnormality is a lethal one, then expectant management is reasonable. However, the patient should be counseled about the risk and implications to the normal twin if the abnormal cotwin dies in utero.
- The risks of TTTS and discordant fetal growth restriction are still present, regardless of the anatomical malformation, and the patient should be advised of this. For some anomalies (anencephaly), which can result in significant polyhydramnios and preterm labor, earlier intervention may be required.
- As with a singleton pregnancy, all options should be discussed, including selective termination or termination of the entire pregnancy.
- Unlike dichorionic placentation, the monochorionic placenta contains numerous vascular anastomoses. These anastomoses preclude the injection of a lethal agent into the affected twin's vasculature as a method of feticide. Additionally, there is the risk of agonal intertwin transfusion at the time of fetal demise and serious sequelae to its cotwin. An ablative technique occluding both the artery and vein of the abnormal twin is required.
- Earlier in gestation, radiofrequency, interstitial laser, and fetoscopic techniques have been described. Radiofrequency and interstitial laser are ultrasound guided procedures with fewer complications suitable at gestations <16 weeks.
- Bipolar diathermy cord occlusion is a relatively simple technique, which can be performed at mid gestation through a single port under ultrasound control with good results. Membrane rupture complicates up to 20% of cord occlusion cases. This procedure becomes technically difficult to perform (due to increasing cord thickness) beyond 28 weeks' gestation. Fetoscopic techniques have also been described, although complication rates are higher.
- Cord ligation may be an option at later gestations, although this can be technically very challenging.

Monochorionic twins discordant for growth restriction
- Growth restriction can complicate up to 40% of monochorionic twin pregnancies. TTTS can mimic some features of discordant growth, such as a small fetus, oligohydramnios, and abnormal umbilical artery Dopplers. However, discordant growth can be distinguished from TTTS by the lack of recipient phenotypic features, particularly polyhydramnios and an enlarged bladder in the larger twin.
- In monochorionic twins, the availability of oxygen and nutrient supply are related to the degree of placental sharing, the quality of implantation of each placental portion, and the angioarchitecture of the placental mass. Unequal placental sharing is a significant risk factor for birth weight discordance in monochorionic twins.
- Velamentous cord insertion occurs in 65% of monochorionic placentae compared with only 18% of dichorionic placentae. Birth weight discordancy correlates with placental territory discordancy and the degree of balance in arteriovenous anastomoses.

- Close monitoring in a fetal medicine unit is essential with weekly or biweekly assessment of fetal well-being. Umbilical artery Dopplers may not have the same prognostic importance as in singleton pregnancies because the presence of an arterial–arterial anastomosis can influence the waveform.
- Additional criteria of fetal well-being (liquor volume, ductus venosus, and middle cerebral artery Dopplers, fetal activity, and breathing movements) must be incorporated into the monitoring algorithm.
- Management options depend on the gestational age. A severely growth restricted cotwin of a previable weight and gestation may well warrant selective termination. If gestation is sufficiently advanced, delivery may be an option, although this usually means subjecting both fetuses to problems of prematurity.
- Some investigators have suggested that fetocopic laser therapy to "dichorionize" the placenta by ablating all vessels crossing the intertwin membrane may help protect the cotwin in the event of demise of the growth restricted fetus. This, however, cannot prevent agonal transfusion due to deep placental anastomoses.

Monochorionic monoamniotic twins
- Monochorionic monoamniotic twins occur in 1%–2% of monozygous conceptions and result if cellular division takes place 7–14 days after fertilization.
- There is a high incidence (71%) of cord entanglement (Figs. 15.6 and 15.7) often from the first trimester with more than 50% of perinatal deaths due to this complication.

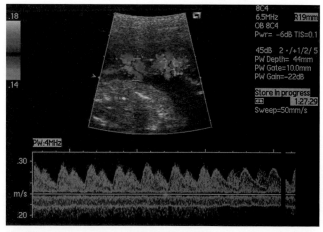

Fig. 15.6. Doppler waveform of cord entanglement showing two asynchronous arterial waveforms. See color plate section.

15

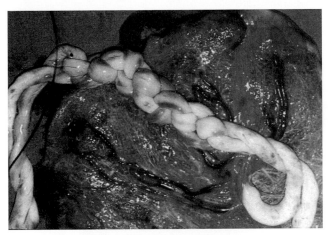

Fig. 15.7. Cord entanglement in monoamniotic twins.

- There is no agreed protocol for monitoring or management of these pregnancies. Prevention of cord entanglement is largely unpreventable as it occurs from very early in pregnancy. There is evidence that the perinatal loss rate increases significantly beyond 32 weeks, which would support elective delivery after maternal corticosteroids at this gestation.
- Another approach would be to use maternal sulindac (selective COX2 inhibitor) therapy (200 mg twice daily from 20 weeks) to reduce amniotic fluid volume, thereby limiting fetal movements and the risk of fatal cord tightening. Sulindac has minimal effect on ductus arteriosus closure prior to 32 weeks. Perinatal survival rates of 100% have been reported with this management.
- Delivery by cesarean section is advisable due to the increased risk of intrapartum cord accidents.

Acardiac twin
- Acardiac malformation, also known as the twin reversed arterial perfusion (TRAP) sequence, is characterized by lack of cardiac development associated with a spectrum of malformations and reduction anomalies (Fig. 15.8).
- One-third occur in monochorionic monoamniotic pregnancies and the remainder in monochorionic diamniotic conceptions.
- The acardiac fetus is perfused in a paradoxical retrograde fashion by a structurally normal "pump" twin through a single artery-to-artery anastomosis. Alternatively, the single umbilical artery of the acardiac twin can connect directly with the umbilical cord of the pump twin.
- The acardiac twin therefore lacks a functional placenta and its entire fetoplacental blood volume is confined to its own vascular tree.

15

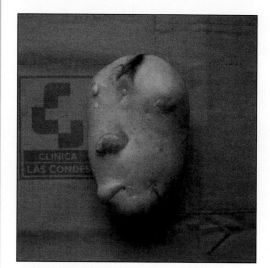

Fig. 15.8. Acardiac fetus.

- It is a very rare condition, occurring with an incidence of 1 in 35 000 deliveries, 1 in 100 monozygotic twins, and 1 in 30 monozygotic triplets.
- The size of the acardiac fetus can vary from a small amorphous structure to more than double the size of its cotwin. The heart may be completely absent (holoacardia) or be in a primitive state of development (pseudoacardia).
- The diagnosis is made on ultrasound by the classic absence of identifiable cardiac pulsations and abnormal formation of the head, trunk, and upper extremities. The lower limbs, although malformed, often show better definition and may show some movements.
- There are usually marked tissue edema and abnormal cystic areas in the upper part of the body of the acardiac twin. A two-vessel cord is present in more than two-thirds of cases. Polyhydramnios in the acardiac twin's sac develops if there is a functioning renal system. Occasionally, the rudimentary heart may demonstrate cardiac pulsations.
- The main risk to the pregnancy is the continuous growth of the acardiac twin and the associated "vascular steal" phenomenon, which leads to cardiac failure, polyhydramnios and even death of the pump twin. Untreated, the perinatal mortality rate approaches 55%.
- The size of the acardiac twin and the cardiovascular status of the pump twin are the most important factors to predict pump twin outcome and guide management.
- An increase in size of the acardiac twin on serial ultrasound scans is another poor prognostic factor. An enlarging acardiac twin suggests an increase in cardiac demand of the pump twin. Conversely, a

15

decrease in size may suggest a reduction of blood flow to the acardiac twin that may result in spontaneous resolution of the condition.

- The goal of treatment is to prevent cardiac failure in the pump twin. The dilemma is identifying the appropriate case for treatment. If the pump twin is hydropic or shows clear evidence of increased cardiac dysfunction, then urgent treatment is required.
- If there is no evidence of pump twin compromise, expectant management is an option as some series have shown almost 90% perinatal survival. Others have recommended using the acardiac to pump twin's abdominal circumference ratio to help decide management.
- If the ratio is greater than 50% at presentation, then intervention is indicated. If the ratio is les then 50%, expectant management is reasonable. If, however, there is evidence of pump twin cardiovascular dysfunction, intervention is again indicated.
- There are many treatment methods that have been described. Broadly, they can be divided into cord occlusion or intrafetal ablation techniques. The disadvantage of cord occlusion techniques is the technical challenge posed by the very short cord of the acardiac twin, which is in close proximity to the pump twin. An intrafetal approach targets the aorta or pelvic vessels of the acardiac twin.
- Both fetoscopic and ultrasound guided procedures have been described, including radiofrequency ablation of the acardiac twin, interstitial laser, injection of sclerosants, monopolar diathermy, etc. In small series, survival rates as high as 90% at term have been reported.

Conjoint twins
- Conjoint twins have an incidence of 1 in 200 monozygous conceptions. Classification is based on the site of fusion: inferior conjunction (diprosopus, dicephalus, ischiopagus, pygopagus), superior conjunction (dipygus, syncephalus, craniopagus) mid-conjunction (thoracopagus, omphalopagus, rachipagus). The site and the extent of fusion are extremely variable, the most common form being thoracopagus (70%).
- Prognosis depends on the degree and site of fusion, the extent of shared organs, and the presence of additional anomalies.
- Management in a tertiary center with facilities for prenatal imaging and postnatal surgery is essential. Parents need to be counseled at length about the outcome and the complexity of some of the surgical procedures and the morbidity involved. Termination of pregnancy should be discussed for the more complex cases with very poor prognosis.
- Surgical outcome appears in part, to be, related to whether separation was performed electively or as an emergency procedure. Survival rates of 80% in elective cases compared with 28% for emergency surgery have been reported. Emergency procedures not only preclude optimal multidisciplinary surgical preparation, but are also associated with deterioration in the condition of one or both babies, leading to poorer outcomes.

MONOCHORIONIC TWINS

LIQUOR VOLUME ABNORMALITIES

Amniotic fluid

- There is a wide variation in amniotic fluid volume throughout gestation, with a gradual increase as pregnancy progresses before decreasing after 36 weeks' gestation.
- Amniotic fluid volume is the net result between inflow and outflow of fluid into the amniotic cavity. In early gestation the most likely source of amniotic fluid is active transport of solute by the amnion into the amniotic space with water moving passively along.
- Later in pregnancy, fetal urine, secretions from the respiratory tract, transfer of fluid across the chorionic plate and umbilical cord (intramembranous flow), and movement of fluid directly between the amniotic cavity and maternal blood across the wall of the uterus (transmembranous flow) all contribute to amniotic fluid volume.
- Fetal urine is present in the amniotic space as early as 8–11 weeks' gestation, but is the major contributor of amniotic fluid only later in pregnancy. At term, fetal urine flow may be as much as 1000–1200 ml/day.
- Any condition that prevents either the formation of urine (renal agenesis, renal dysplasia) or its egress into the amniotic sac (bladder outlet obstruction, fetal growth restriction) will cause oligohydramnios.
- Any condition that causes increased fetal urine production (maternal diabetes) may cause polyhydramnios.
- Fetal swallowing plays an important role in maintaining amniotic fluid volume during the latter half of the pregnancy. Obstruction to the upper gastrointestinal tract (esophageal atresia, duodenal atresia) or any condition that impairs fetal swallowing will result in polyhydramnios. Table 16.1 shows the various contributions to the inflow and outflow of amniotic fluid in the human fetus.
- In the first trimester, amniotic fluid has an electrolyte composition and osmolality similar to that of fetal and maternal blood. As fetal urine begins to enter the amniotic cavity, amniotic fluid osmolality decreases compared with fetal blood.
- Near term, the amniotic fluid osmolality is lowest (250–260 mOsm/kg water) compared with fetal blood osmolality of 280 mOsm/kg water. This low osmolality is a result of extremely hypotonic fetal urine (60–140 mOsm/kg water) in combination with a lesser volume of isotonic lung fluid.
- Amniotic fluid volume can be assessed either qualitatively or quantitatively. The amniotic fluid index (AFI) (normal range 5–25 cm) is the sum of the deepest pockets of amniotic fluid in four quadrants of the uterine cavity. The deepest vertical pool of liquor measurement is an alternative method of assessing liquor volume. Neither method has convincingly been judged superior to the other.
- Oligohhydramnios has been variously defined as an AFI less than 5 cm (standard definition) or less than 8 cm (alternate definition), and

Table 16.1 *Daily amniotic fluid dynamics in the human fetus*

Inflow	Outflow
Urine flow (1000–1200 ml)	Swallowing (500–1000 ml)
Lung fluid (340 ml) (50% swallowed)	Intramembranous (200–500 ml)
Pharyngeal fluid (10 ml)	Transmembranous (10 ml)

16

polyhydramnios as greater than 25 cm (standard definition) or greater then 18 cm (alternate definition). A deepest pool of 8 cm indicates excess liquor, whereas a deepest pool of <2 cm suggest oligohydramnios.

Oligohydramnios

- Any condition that reduces fetal urine production or obstruction to the lower urinary tract will cause oligohydramnios.
- Causes of oligohydramnios include ruptured membranes, maternal ingestion of medication (indomethacin, angiotensin converting enzyme inhibitors), congenital malformations, aneuploidy, fetal growth restriction, etc.
- The incidence of oligohydramnios is difficult to ascertain, but is believed to complicate up to 8% of all pregnancies.
- Once oligohydramnios is suspected subjectively, the AFI or the deepest vertical pool should be measured. Careful examination of the fetal anatomy should be performed to exclude a structural malformation as a cause of the oligohydramnios. Abnormalities in the renal system (bilateral multicystic dysplastic kidney, renal agenesis, lower urinary tract obstruction) must be excluded. Color/power Doppler of renal arteries excludes renal agenesis without need for amnioinfusion.
- Fetal growth and comprehensive fetal Doppler assessment should be carried out to exclude intrauterine growth restriction.
- If there is severe oligohydramnios mid gestation during the critical period of pulmonary development, there is a significant risk of pulmonary hypoplasia. The patient will need to be counseled that, even if the pregnancy progresses to term, the perinatal outcome may be very poor. A deepest vertical pool of <1 cm is associated with a 90% risk of perinatal mortality due to pulmonary hypoplasia.
- Severe oligohydramnios/anhydramnios can result in structural malformations and contractures of the extremities (talipes) or the Potter's sequence.
- Amnioinfusion may be necessary to improve visualization of the fetus and permit karyotyping to be performed.

16

- The perinatal prognosis depends on the cause of the oligohydramnios. In preterm rupture of membranes, the prognosis may be very poor due to the risk of prematurity and infection. A thoraco-abdominal ratio <0.8 after 26 weeks suggests pulmonary hypoplasia.
- Serial amnioinfusion may have a role to restore amniotic fluid volume but this is only applicable in a few select cases. The cumulative procedure-related risk is not insignificant.
- Termination of pregnancy should be offered for bilateral renal agenesis/multicystic kidneys, aneuploidy, severe early onset growth restriction or severe oligohydramnios with onset <23 weeks' gestation.
- Oligohydramnios (AFI <5 cm or deepest pool <2 cm) may be associated with increased fetal distress, meconium staining of liquor, need for emergency cesarean section, low Apgar scores, and abnormal umbilical cord pH. The evidence for adverse intrapartum problems is not strong, with many publications suggesting only a weak association.
- The risk for recurrence will depend on the underlying cause.

Polyhydramnios

- Polyhydramnios is defined as an AFI >25 cm or a deepest vertical pool of >8 cm (Fig. 16.1). Between 50% and 60% of cases have no obvious cause (idiopathic). Other major causes include poorly controlled maternal diabetes mellitus, fetal structural malformations, and multiple pregnancy.

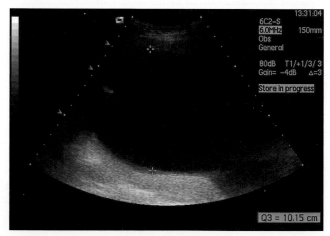

Fig. 16.1. Polyhydramnios (deepest pool greater than 8 cm).

16

- Fetal malformations associated with polyhydramnios include pharyngeal/esophageal obstruction, upper small bowel obstruction (duodenal or jejunal atresia), open neural tube defects, neuromuscular disorders (myotonic dystrophy), cardiac abnormalities, tumors, vascular malformations (vein of Galen aneurysm), infections, skeletal dysplasias, etc.
- Aneuploidy is present in up to 10% of fetuses with malformations and in 1% when the polyhydramnios is isolated. In persistent polyhydramnios, the risk of aneuploidy is increased (10%–20%) compared with polyhydramnios that resolves.
- Once polyhydramnios is detected subjectively, an objective (AFI or deepest pool) assessment of the amniotic fluid volume should be performed. A detailed maternal history should be obtained. Maternal diabetes should be excluded. A family history of myotonic dystrophy or past history of skeletal dysplasia/arthrogryposis should be excluded.
- An assessment of the severity of the poyhydramnios should be made. The fetus should be carefully examined to exclude a structural malformation. The presence of a fetal stomach does not necessarily exclude high intestinal obstruction. A double bubble appearance in the fetal abdomen may suggest duodenal atresia.
- Aneuploidy risk depends on the underlying cause, presence of associated structural anomalies, and the degree of excess liquor. Karyotyping for isolated mild polyhydramnios is controversial.
- Amnioreduction should be performed if the AFI is >40 cm or if the patient is symptomatic. Treatment of the polyhydramnios will depend on the underlying cause (anti-arrhythmic therapy for fetal supraventicular tachycardia, pleuro-amniotic shunting if pleural effusions, correction of fetal anemia, etc.).
- Maternal medical therapy using cyclooxygenase inhibitors (indomethacin, sulindac) is an option particularly in unexplained cases. Therapy should be discontinued beyond 30–32 weeks because of the risk of ductus arteriosus closure in the fetus.
- Termination of pregnancy should be offered for aneuploidy, lethal anomalies, and major malformations. Counseling by a pediatric surgeon is helpful if a surgical cause is felt likely.
- The patient should be counseled about the risks of preterm labor, malpresentation and cord prolapse. Active delivery by 38 weeks is reasonable in view of the increased risk of unexplained stillbirth. There is 2–5× increased risk of perinatal mortality.
- The neonatologists should be informed about the risk of upper gastrointestinal tract obstruction. Esophageal atresia is easily diagnosed by the inability to pass a nasogastric tube.

INFECTIONS

- Many infections during pregnancy can carry a risk for intrauterine transmission, which may result in fetal damage. Some agents are teratogenic, while others cause fetal or neonatal diseases of varying severity.
- The ability of infectious agents to cross the placenta and infect the fetus depends on many factors including the maternal immune status. Primary infections during pregnancy are much more damaging than secondary infections or reactivations.
- The fetal phenotype depends on the gestation at which the infection occurs. In general, infections in the first trimester are more likely to cause major structural malformations compared with infections later in pregnancy. Placental and intrafetal calcifications may be seen (Figs. 17.1 and 17.2).

Parvovirus (erythema infectiosum)

- Parvovirus B19 is a highly infectious DNA virus that tends to occur in mini epidemics. The virus is spread by respiratory droplets, by blood products especially pooled factor XIII and IX concentrates and transplacentally during pregnancy.
- Parvovirus B19 infection is common in childhood, continues at a low rate throughout adult life and, by the time adults are in their 50–60s, most are sero positive. The peak incidence of erythema infectiosum is in late winter and early spring.
- Following infection, immunoglobulins IgM, IgG and IgA are produced. One week after the infection, a mild illness develops (pyrexia, malaise, myalgia, and itchiness). The main immune response at this stage is production of IgM. IgM rises at 10–12 days postinfection and peaks when the viral load is highest. IgM can persist for about 3 months from the primary illness.
- A second phase of symptoms develops about 17–18 days after the infection (rash, itchiness, or arthralgia). After about 10–14 days, IgG is produced and immunity is then life-long. IgA is detected in about 90% of infected cases and is postulated to protect against infection by the nasopharyngeal route.
- The P antigen on the red blood cell is a cellular receptor of the virus. 1 in 100 000 humans are P negative and are therefore resistant to Parvovirus B19 infection. Parvovirus B19 inhibits erythroid cell differentiation and is cytotoxic for erythroid precursor cells. Direct toxic cell injury, cytolytic destruction, or apotosis may be responsible for erythroid aplasia in high-risk patients.
- Parvovirus B19 can be detected by isolation of viral DNA by direct hybridization or by PCR. Maternal serology is reliable to detect a current or recent infection. IgG avidity studies can be used to diagnose an acute infection. Low IgG avidity will be found early.

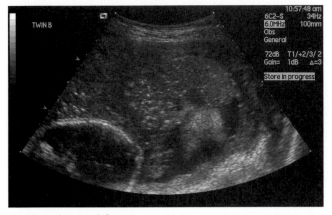

Fig. 17.1. Placenta calcifications.

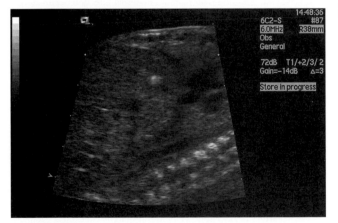

Fig. 17.2. Fetal liver calcifications.

- Aymptomatic sero conversion following viremia is common in both children and adults. Erythema infectiosum (fifth disease) is the most common clinical manifestation in childhood. A rash, mainly on the cheeks, is typical. The rash is likely due to the formation and deposition of immune complexes in the skin.

- Arthropathy is the most common manifestation of infection in adults. 60% of adult females are affected, compared to 30% of adult males and 10% of children. The symptoms coincide with the appearance of circulating antibodies.
- Various hematological/immunological aberrations can occur: thrombocytopenia, transient aplastic anemia/red cell aplasia, and virus-associated hemophagocytic syndrome (VAHS) have all been reported. Additional complications include meningoencephalitis, myocarditis, vasculitis, hepatitis, and liver failure. Immunocompromised patients are particularly at risk and should be monitored carefully.
- Infection during pregnancy can cause several problems: fetal anemia, non-immune hydrops, miscarriage, preterm labor, and intrauterine death across all gestations.
- Fetal abnormalities associated with Parvovirus B19 are rare and there is no evidence that Parvovirus B19 is a significant teratogen.
- Risk assessment for maternal infection during pregnancy is especially important during epidemics. Most women are already immune to Parvovirus B19 prior to pregnancy.
- Transplacental transmission of the virus can occur in 30% of infected pregnant women. The fetus is at greatest risk for an adverse outcome between 3 and 6 weeks following maternal infection. The risk of adverse fetal outcome is increased if maternal infection occurs during the first two trimesters of pregnancy.
- Parvovirus B19 infects the liver, which is the main site of erythrocyte production in the fetus. In the second trimester, when the liver is the main source of hematopoetic activity and the half-life of red cells is short, the fetus is more at risk.
- Severe fetal anemia can lead to cardiac failure and non-immune hydrops. Direct viral infection of myocardiocytes causes myocarditis and worsens the heart failure and hydrops. These fetuses are at particular risk of intrauterine death.
- The risk of fetal complications depends mainly on the gestational age at the time of maternal infection. The highest risk for fetal loss is during 9–16 weeks' gestation. Fetal sequelae are rare in the last 8 weeks of pregnancy. Hydrops has been reported between 1 and 20 weeks after maternal infection. Usually, it becomes evident after 3–4 weeks.
- If a patient has serological evidence of infection during pregnancy, the fetus should be monitored with weekly ultrasound scans. Middle cerebral artery peak systolic velocities should be checked at each visit to detect the development of fetal anemia. Hydrops is almost always due to severe fetal anemia.
- Intrauterine transfusions correct the anemia and lead to resolution of the hydrops. Survival rates >80% have been reported. Some hydropic fetuses may be thrombocytopenic, but platelet transfusions are usually not required. Intrafetal bleeding is rare.
- There are no long-term neurodevelopmental issues. Congenital anemia may be due to persistence of the parvovirus infection in the bone marrow.

- If fetal anemia develops, most cases will require only one transfusion.
- Mode of delivery is on standard obstetric grounds. The baby should be monitored postdelivery for signs on ongoing anemia.

17

Cytomegalovirus (CMV)

- CMV is a double-stranded DNA virus belonging to the herpes virus family, which has the capacity to establish life-long latency in the host. Transmission is by close contact between individuals, although contamination from urine, saliva, semen, cervical secretions, and breast milk can also occur.
- CMV infections are endemic and lack seasonal variation. The incidence of congenital CMV infection varies between 0.2% and 2%. The most important risk factor for maternal CMV infection during pregnancy is frequent and prolonged exposure to young children. Children less than 2 years of age excrete the virus in both saliva and urine for approximately 2 years.
- Congenital infection occurs when a primary CMV infection develops during or just before pregnancy. The rate of vertical transmission increases as gestation progresses, but the severity is greatest if it develops early in pregnancy. There is indirect evidence that re-infection of seropositive patients with new strains of CMV can occur.
- Primary CMV infections are reported in 1%–4% of seronegative women during pregnancy and the risk for fetal transmission is 30%–40%. Reactivation of a CMV infection during pregnancy occurs in 10%–30% of seropositive women with a transmission risk of 1%–3%.
- Both maternal cellular and humoral immunity mitigate viral transmission during pregnancy. Patients with impaired cellular immunity (HIV, immunosuppressive therapy) are more likely to transmit the virus to the fetus. The presence of CMV IgG is inversely correlated with vertical transmission. It is presumed that, in recurrent infections, pre-existing immunity reduces or eliminates maternal viremia and is protective to the fetus.
- The best method for the serologic diagnosis of asymptomatic maternal primary infection is seroconversion. IgM antibodies to CMV develop in all primary infections but may also occur after reactivation or re-infection and remain present for several months.
- The presence of IgM is therefore not definitive for a primary CMV infection (unless seroconversion can be demonstrated). Antibody avidity is a better method to time the infection. Avidity increases in the first weeks and months after a primary infection.
- The combination of anti-CMV IgM and low-avidity anti-CMV IgG is the best way to diagnose a primary maternal infection. Examination of amniotic fluid or fetal blood may be a helpful adjunct in prenatal diagnosis. Although viral culture of the amniotic fluid is 100% specific, it often yields false-negative results.
- Amniotic fluid PCR for CMV DNA, especially after 21 weeks' gestation is sensitive and specific for fetal infection. A positive result, however, does not mean that the fetus will be affected. The presence

17

of fetal or placental abnormalities on ultrasound is more predictive of disease and long-term consequences.

- Ultrasound features include hydrops, ventriculomegaly, microcephaly, intrauterine growth restriction, ascites, pyelectasis, megaloureter, and periventricular or hepatic and intestinal calcifications. An increase in placental thickness is also a marker for congenital infection.
- About 10% of infants with congenital CMV infection have signs and symptoms at birth, but 90% are asymptomatic. Jaundice, hepatosplenomegaly and petechiae in a growth-restricted preterm baby should raise suspicions of a congenital viral infection and hence trigger testing.
- Severely affected babies have a mortality rate of 30%. Death is usually due to hepatic dysfunction, bleeding, disseminated intravascular coagulation, or secondary bacterial infections superimposed on the complications of prematurity.
- Long-term disabilities include severe developmental delay, autism, learning disabilities, cerebral palsy, epilepsy, hearing, and visual impairment.
- Congenital CMV infection is the single most important cause of sensorineural hearing loss or deafness in childhood. Hearing loss occurs in 10%–15% of all infants with congenital CMV with much higher rates if there was evidence of neonatal infection.
- Visual impairment and strabismus are common in children with clinically apparent CMV infection and can be caused by chorioretinitis, pigmentary retinitis, macular scarring, optic atrophy, and central cortical defects. The incidence of chorioretinitis in symptomatic neonates is between 15% and 30%.
- If the diagnosis is confirmed antenatally and if there are ultrasound abnormalities present, the significant risk of long-term problems should be discussed with the parents. If infection has occurred early in pregnancy, the prognosis is particularly grim because of the increased severity of the congenital infection. The option of termination of pregnancy should be discussed.
- There is no effective antenatal treatment. Hyperimmune globulin therapy has been used in some cases with reasonable results, but this is not in mainstream practice yet.
- Ganciclovir has been used to treat neonates with congenital infection.

Toxoplasmosis

- *Toxoplasma gondii* is an obligate intracellular protozoan that can infect all mammals, who serve as intermediate hosts. Eating raw or undercooked meat and meat products, poor kitchen hygiene, contact with cat litter, and eating unwashed raw vegetables or fruits is associated with an increased risk of infection.
- 90% of infections are asymptomatic. If symptomatic, a low-grade fever, malaise, headache, and cervical lymphadenopathy can be present. More severe complications (encephalitis, myocarditis, hepatitis, pneumonia) are rare but can complicate acute disease.

17

- Transplacental spread during a primary attack can cause congenital toxoplasmosis. The incidence of maternal primary infection is relatively low, with seroconversion rates ranging from 0.2%–0.5%.
- Congenital toxoplasmosis can include a wide range of manifestations, ranging from mild chorioretinitis, which can present many years after birth, to miscarriage, neurodevelopmental delay, microcephaly, hydrocephalus, and seizures.
- Congenital infection occurs in 20% of offspring after primary infection. Transmission rates increase with gestation (<5% in the first months of pregnancy to approximately 80% in the third trimester). The later in pregnancy that congenital infection occurs, the less severe the consequences are to the fetus.
- In asymptomatic women, the only sign of primary infection during pregnancy is seroconversion (i.e. detection of IgG or IgM). IgG levels become detectable 1–2 weeks after infection and remain elevated indefinitely, while IgM levels increase rapidly within days and remain elevated for up to 2–3 months.
- In 7% of women IgM levels can remain positive for >2 years making timing of infection difficult.
- IgG avidity studies may help with the diagnosis (low avidity <30% indicates recent infection within 3 months, high avidity >40% indicates infection >6 months previously).
- If primary maternal infection has been confirmed, evidence of fetal infection should be obtained. Fetal blood sampling or amniocentesis for *T. gondii* DNA PCR is very sensitive and indicates fetal infection.
- Fetal sequelae are very likely if abnormalities (intracerebral calcifications, ventriculomegaly) are present on ultrasound scan. Termination of pregnancy should be offered. In pregnancies that continue, serial scans should be arranged.
- If maternal infection is diagnosed, it is not known if antenatal treatment is effective. A systematic review of non-randomized studies found therapy to be effective in five trials but ineffective in four studies.
- It is currently recommended that all pregnant women who have been diagnosed with a primary infection be treated antenatally with spiramycin +/− pyrimethamine-sulfadiazine. Pyrimethamine is teratogenic and contraindicated in the first trimester.
- Detection of IgM or IgA antibodies in an infant is highly sensitive for the diagnosis of congenital toxoplasmosis. If an infant is diagnosed with congenital toxoplasmosis, recommendations include treatment with pyrimethamine, sulfadiazine, and leucovorin for up to 1 year.

Rubella

- The rubella virus is an RNA virus, which can cause severe fetal consequences if primary infection occurs during pregnancy. Humans are the only known natural hosts, and transmission occurs by aerosol droplets via the respiratory tract. The virus replicates primarily in the nasopharynx and viremia begins 5 to 7 days postinfection.

17

- Rubella is usually a mild infection in children, but may be more severe in adults. Up to 20%–25% of infections may be subclinical. Primary prevention is possible with preconception vaccination.
- The risk of congenital rubella syndrome is greatest if infection occurs earlier in pregnancy. There is a >80% risk of congenital defects if rubella is acquired in the first 12 weeks of pregnancy.
- Maternal re-infection can occur and poses a risk to the fetus, although substantially less compared with a primary attack. Re-infection is indicated by a significant rise in rubella IgG antibodies, sometimes to very high levels, in a woman with pre-existing antibodies.
- Congenital infection occurs in 8%, but the risk of defects is usually <5% when reinfection occurs. No congenital defects have been reported when maternal re-infection has occurred after 12 weeks' gestation. Re-infection tends to occur in women with low antibody titers.
- If infection occurs just prior to conception or in the first trimester, ocular defects, cardiovascular malformations (patent ductus arteriosus, pulmonary stenosis), severe fetal growth restriction, and deafness are common manifestations.
- Second trimester infections tend to cause deafness, retinitis, microcephaly, and neurodevelopmental delay.
- Third trimester infection results in fetal growth restriction, although there is significant overlay in the fetal manifestations throughout gestation.
- Rubella vaccines are contraindicated in pregnancy (3% risk of fetal infection), but inadvertent vaccination in pregnancy is not an indication for termination of pregnancy or prenatal diagnosis.
- Because of the considerable similarity in the clinical features of a primary rubella infection and various other viral infections, laboratory testing should always be performed.
- Acute rubella infection is characterized by a progressive rise in antibody titers. Rubella-specific IgM become detectable about 5 days after the maternal rash and can persist for about 6 weeks. False-positive results can occur in patients with parvovirus or mononucleosis infections, or in those with a positive rheumatoid factor.
- For a more precise diagnosis and timing of the infection, IgG avidity studies are important. IgG antibody avidity appears and increases during the first 3 months after the onset of the rash. A low avidity index is generally observed up to 6 weeks after the primary infection.
- Invasive prenatal diagnosis is most valuable when primary rubella cannot be excluded in the first trimester due to equivocal rubella IgM results, when there is laboratory confirmation of primary rubella during 12–18 weeks' gestation or when rubella re-infection occurs before 12 weeks' gestation.
- Chorionic villus, amniotic fluid, and fetal blood samples can all be used for prenatal diagnosis. Fetal blood can also be tested for rubella IgM. Samples should be obtained 7–8 weeks after primary maternal infection and after the 21st week of gestation.
- Parents should be counseled that fetal infection is not always accompanied by congenital defects.

17

- No antiviral drug is available to treat rubella or prevent transmission to the fetus. Human normal immunoglobulin or rubella hyperimmune globulin soon after exposure may reduce the amount of viremia and fetal damage.
- The incidence of fetal infection does not seem to be reduced with maternal therapy and follow-up is required. Immunoglobulin prophylaxis is recommended only for rubella-exposed women in early pregnancy for whom termination is not an option.
- If the primary maternal infection has occurred in the first trimester, or if fetal infection is confirmed on invasive testing, or if ultrasound abnormalities are present, parents should be counseled about the significant risk of congenital infection and offered termination of pregnancy.

INFECTIONS

RED CELL AND PLATELET ALLOIMMUNIZATION

Red cell alloimmunization

- Pregnancies complicated by red cell alloimmunization may result in fetal anemia (hemolytic disease of the newborn) secondary to transplacental passage of maternal IgG, which causes progressive fetal hemolysis.
- It can range in severity from being detectable only in laboratory tests through to severe fetal anaemia resulting in hydrops, stillbirth, or the birth of babies with severe anemia and jaundice.
- Antibodies that can cause fetal hemolysis include anti-D, anti-Kell, anti-c, and anti-E, although the risk may be present albeit to a lesser degree with some of the other red cell antibodies.
- Once alloimmunization has occurred and the fetus is at risk of anemia, the principles of management are similar, regardless of the type of antibody involved.
- However, in Kell alloimmunization caution is required as antibody levels do not always correlate with disease severity. With this antibody, there is greater suppression of erythropoiesis rather than intravascular hemolysis and neonatal jaundice is less of a problem.
- The incidence of anti-D alloimmunization has decreased significantly with the advent of both antenatal and postnatal prophylaxis. Anti-D prophylaxis should be administered after any sensitizing event and, if the fetomaternal hemorrhage is suspected to be large, quantification of the hemorrhage should be performed to assess the need for further anti-D prophylaxis.
- Sensitizing events include threatened miscarriage, ectopic pregnancy, any invasive prenatal procedure (chorionic villous sampling, amniocentesis, etc.), antepartum hemorrhage, external cephalic version, closed abdominal injury, and intrauterine injury.
- The National Institute for Health and Clinical Excellence (NICE) currently recommends two doses of anti-D immunoglobulin (500 IU) antenatally at 28 and 34 weeks' gestation to non-sensitized RhD-negative women.
- Patients who are weakly RhD positive (previously Du positive) have a quantitative rather than a qualitative difference in the D antigen and are not at risk of RhD alloimmunization. They do not require prophylaxis with anti-D immunoglobulin.
- The most important cause of anti-D antibodies now is immunization during pregnancy, when no overt sensitizing event has occurred. Late immunization during a first pregnancy is responsible for 18%–27% of cases. Immunization during a second or subsequent pregnancy probably accounts for a similar proportion of cases, although it is often impossible to distinguish late sensitization from failure of prophylaxis at the end of the preceding pregnancy.
- The cause of the alloimmunization should be ascertained (inadequate prophylaxis, administrative failure, blood transfusion, etc.). Details of

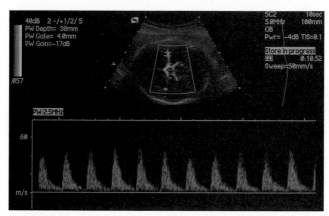

Fig. 18.1. Middle cerebral artery peak systolic velocity. See color plate section.

previously affected pregnancies – particularly in utero transfusions, neonatal anemia, and the need for exchange transfusions or photo-therapy should also be obtained. This information enables a risk assessment/profile of the pregnancy to be made.

- Once alloimmunization has occurred, the fetus is at risk from anaemia, and the risk appears to increase with increasing concentrations. In the UK and Europe, a threshold value of 15 IU/ml has been recommended for invasive testing, as only mild hemolytic disease is noted with anti-D levels below this value.
- Once alloimmunization is detected and, if the antibody titers are rising, referral to a fetal medicine unit should be made. Paternal genotype should be ascertained – if the father is homozygous for the red cell antigen, then all pregnancies are potentially at risk.
- It is now possible to check the fetal genotype non-invasively from maternal blood. Using polymerase chain reaction techniques, fetal RhD status can be detected with 100% sensitivity using fetal DNA extracted from maternal plasma. This technique is sensitive enough to detect the RhD gene in a single cell. The fetal Kell and c genotype can also be detected using this method.
- If the fetus is RhD positive, then it will be at risk for anemia and the pregnancy needs to be serially monitored. Pregnancies at risk should be monitored on a weekly basis, looking specifically at the middle cerebral artery peak systolic velocity (Fig. 18.1). Other signs that might suggest fetal anemia include polyhydramnios, skin edema, and cardiomegaly.
- Peak systolic velocities greater than 1.5 multiples of the median (MoM) for the specific gestation are predictive of moderate or severe fetal anaemia, with 100% sensitivity and a false-positive rate of 12%. This method of monitoring should be used with caution after 36 weeks as the sensitivity decreases.

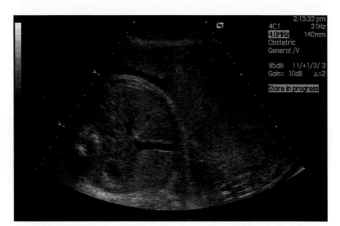

Fig. 18.2. Fetal blood sampling and transfusion at the intrahepatic vein.

- Doppler ultrasonography of the middle cerebral artery correlates well with increasing levels of bilirubin in the amniotic fluid. This non-invasive method has superseded the traditional technique of serial amniocentesis for the spectral analysis of amniotic fluid at 450 nm ($\Box$OD450), first described by Liley in 1961.
- If monitoring of the middle cerebral artery indicates anemia, fetal blood sampling (FBS) and intrauterine transfusion (IUT) are indicated (Fig. 18.2). The patient should be counseled that the loss rate related to the procedure depends on the gestation, site of sampling, and underlying pathology.
- The risk of an uncomplicated FBS is 1%–3%, but if the fetus is hydropic it may be as high as 20%. Fetal blood can be taken either from the placental cord insertion site or from the intrahepatic vein. The intrahepatic approach is less likely to cause fetal distress, but is technically more difficult.
- Complications of FBS include bradycardia, hemorrhage, cord hematoma and tamponade, and fetal death. The procedure is done under continuous ultrasound guidance, and facilities for immediate analysis of the fetal blood should be available.
- Group O negative, cytomegalovirus negative blood that has been cross-matched with a maternal blood sample is used for fetal transfusion. Typically, the donor cells are packed to a volume of 75%–90% to prevent volume overload, and they are irradiated to minimize the risk of graft versus host disease. A final fetal packed cell volume of 45%–55% is desirable post-transfusion.
- The timing of subsequent transfusions is dependent on the rate of decline of the fetal packed cell volume, the presence of hydrops, and gestation. Usually, an interval of 3 to 5 weeks is the norm before the

next transfusion. Weekly middle cerebral artery monitoring is essential. With careful monitoring and appropriate timing of transfusions, delivery should be anticipated at 37–38 weeks' gestation.

- At delivery, cord blood should be collected for analyses of hemoglobin, packed cell volume, and bilirubin, and for a direct antiglobulin test (DAT). The mode of delivery is dependent on standard obstetric grounds.
- Prior intrauterine therapy is not an indication for an elective cesarean section.
- In one review the overall survival was noted to be 84% with non-hydropic fetuses having better outcomes (92%) than hydropic fetuses (70%).
- Newborns may experience on-going anemia. Early anemia is usually the result of passively acquired maternal antibodies causing on-going hemolysis. The criteria for performing exchange transfusions remain controversial, but rapidly rising serum concentrations of bilirubin that are unresponsive to intensive phototherapy are an indication.
- The most common cause of late anemia is a hyporegenerative anemia, usually after several intrauterine transfusions. Affected infants have suppression of erythropoiesis with extremely low reticulocytes, despite a low packed cell volume and normal erythropoietin values. Bone marrow aspirates show erythroid hypoplasia. Top-up transfusions are required only if the infant is symptomatic.
- There is some evidence that the need and frequency of top-up transfusions is decreased if recombinant erythropoietin is used.
- Normal neurodevelopmental outcome occurs in more than 90% of cases. With appropriate management, kernicterus is seen rarely. Sensorineural hearing loss is more common in infants affected by hemolytic disease of the newborn because of the toxic effect of prolonged exposure of bilirubin on the developing eighth cranial nerve.
- Recent studies using maternal intravenous immunoglobulin have shown some benefit in severe cases of RhD incompatibility. The mechanism of action is not clear but may entail downregulation of the maternal immune response, placental antigenic blockade, or antigenic blockade at the level of the fetal reticulo-endothelial system.
- This treatment modality is appropriate only in selected cases (e.g. very early disease). It may prolong the time interval before the first intrauterine treatment is required.

Fetal alloimmune thrombocytopenia
- Fetal and neonatal alloimmune thrombocytopenia are the most common causes of severe thrombocytopenia in fetuses and neonates with an incidence of 1 in 1000 to 1 in 2000 pregnancies.
- Maternal IgG alloantibodies against paternally derived fetal platelet antigens cross the placenta and bind to fetal platelets. The antibody-coated platelets are subsequently removed from the fetal circulation

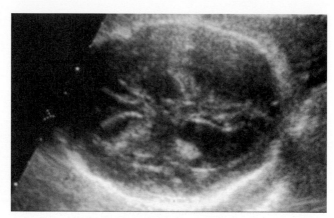

Fig. 18.3. Intracranial hemorrhage and venrticulomegaly.

by the reticuloendothelial system. These same antibodies may also inhibit platelet production. The hemorrhagic sequelae may also be aggravated by endothelial cell damage.

- Platelet alloimmunization is reported in up to 50% of first pregnancies. Fetal platelet antigens are expressed from 16 weeks' gestation, and alloantibody formation with thrombocytopenia may occur as early as 16–20 weeks' gestation.

- To date, there are 16 human platelet-specific antigens (HPA) listed by the Platelet Serology Working Party of the International Society of Blood Transfusion (ISBT). They are numbered in order of their original description and the alleles are labeled alphabetically in the order of their serologic frequency. Each HPA antigen is biallelic and autosomal co-dominant, differing in only one amino acid.

- In Caucasians, HPA-1a is the most common antigen (85%) followed by HPA-5b and HPA-15 incompatibility. In Asians, HPA-4a is the commonest antigen. Unlike HPA-1a alloimmunization, severe thrombocytopenia after HPA-5b incompatibility is rare. The prevalence of HPA-1a negative status is between 1% and 2% in Caucasians.

- The incidence of neonatal thrombocytopenia from various causes is 1%–4%. Thrombocytopenia with an immunological origin is encountered in only 0.3% of the newborns.

- The main complication is intracranial hemorrhage (ICH) (Fig. 18.3) which is associated with major long-term neurological sequelae. 50%–75% of all intracranial bleeding occurs antenatally (14% occurring before 20 weeks and 28% occurring before 30 weeks).

- Untreated newborns are affected by intracranial hemorrhage in 7%–26% of cases with a mortality rate of approximately 7%. Neurological sequelae occur in approximately a fifth of cases.

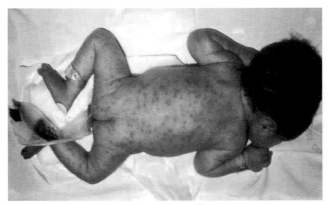

Fig. 18.4. Neonate with severe alloimmnue thrombocytopenia. Note the extensive petechiae.

- ICH has been reported in association with virtually all antigen incompatibilities. In the majority of cases, ICH occurs with platelet counts less than 20×10^9/l, although the risk increases significantly with counts below 50×10^9/l.
- The diagnosis of fetal/neonatal alloimmune thrombocytopenia requires several laboratory observations. There must be HPA incompatibility between mother and child. The presence and identification of maternal anti-platelet alloantibodies is key and these antibodies must be shown to bind to paternal, but not maternal, platelets.
- Good correlation between maternal antibody levels and the severity of disease is lacking, although some studies have shown a higher risk of severe disease with high antibody levels.
- The focus of management is to prevent antenatal or perinatal ICH. The most reliable predictive factor is the presence of a previously affected sibling. If an older sibling had severe disease, subsequent children will be at risk of at least similar severity. Prognostication becomes less reliable if the previously affected sibling only had mild disease.
- The recurrence rate of ICH in a subsequent pregnancy with a previous history of alloimmune thrombocytopenia and ICH is >70%. The risk of ICH following a previous history of alloimmune thrombocytopenia without ICH is estimated to be 7%.
- In the absence of universal screening, most at-risk pregnancies are identified following the birth of a previously affected sibling with thrombocytopenia detected incidently, or clear evidence of bleeding (petechiae) (Fig. 18.4), or ICH.
- Treatment of at-risk pregnancies has evolved with a move away from serial weekly platelet transfusions towards maternal therapy with intravenous immunoglobulin +/− oral steroids. Risk stratification

of the pregnancy is essential. A previously affected pregnancy complicated by fetal/neonatal ICH or severe thrombocytopenia (20×10^9/l) is at highest risk of complications.

- Prior to starting treatment, the fetal genotype should be ascertained. If the father is homozygous for the relevant platelet antigen, there is a 100% risk to all his children. If the father is heterozygous, then there will only be a 50% chance of transmission and therefore of the disease. Fetal genotype can be checked by either CVS or amniocentesis.

- Currently, most centers would commence weekly therapy using maternal intravenous immunoglobulin (IVIG) at 15–16 weeks at a usual dose of 1mg/kg body weight. In selected cases earlier treatment may be indicated. Oral steroids may be used at the very start of therapy or added if there is suboptimal response to maternal immunoglobulin treatment.

- The mode of action of IVIG in alloimmune thrombocytopenia is still unclear. Three possible mechanisms have been postulated. First, dilution of the anti-HPA antibodies in the maternal circulation from the transfused IVIG may result in a lower proportion anti-HPA antibodies among the IgG transferred via the Fc-receptors in the placenta. Second, blockade of the placenta receptor (Fc-R) and decrease in the placental transfer of maternal antibodies (including anti-HPA-antibodies). Third, in the fetus, IVIG may block the Fc-receptors on macrophages and prevent the destruction of anti-body-covered cells.

- Maternal IVIG therapy has a 75% response rate.

- Fetal response to maternal therapy can be checked by performing fetal blood sampling some 6 weeks following initiation of IVIG treatment. There is a significant risk of hemorrhage (6%), even in the hands of experienced operators with a procedure-related mortality rate of >15% if the fetus is thrombocytopenic.

- Intrahepatic vein sampling may have advantages (tamponade from surrounding liver parenchyma) over cordocentesis with less risk of fetal bleeding.

- If there is suboptimum response to maternal therapy, the dose of maternal IVIG can be increased or oral steroids added. In some refractory cases serial platelet transfusions may be required.

- With adequate fetal response, the pregnancy may be allowed to go to term and elective delivery by cesarean section performed. There is increasing evidence that the efficacy of maternal treatment is sufficiently reliable to allow vaginal delivery.

PLACENTA AND UMBILICAL CORD ABNORMALITIES

19

Placenta and umbilical cord

- The human placenta has two components: a large fetal portion that develops from the chorionic sac and a smaller maternal portion derived from the endometrium.
- Development of the placenta depends critically on the differentiation of specialized epithelial cells (cytotrophoblasts) to ensure that the maternal fetal interface allows adequate nutritional supply to the fetus and at the same time elimination of waste products into the maternal circulation. After approximately 6 days postfertilization, the blastocyst implants into the primed endometrium. As soon as implantation takes place, rapid trophoblast proliferation occurs resulting in the formation of two distinct layers: an inner mononuclear (cytotrophoblast) and an outer multinucleated syncytiotrophoblast layer.
- The syncytiotrophoblast produces various lytic enzymes, which enable digit-like processes to invade the endometrial stroma to complete implantation. Initially, the developing embryo obtains its nutrition from glycogen and lipid-laden stromal cells, which degenerate adjacent to the invading syncytiotrophoblast.
- The development of an adequate uteroplacental circulation is critical for the maintenance of the embryo and, by the end of the third postconception week, a basic anatomical system is in place for feto-maternal exchange.
- Lacunar networks, which are filled with maternal blood, form through the fusion of individual syncytiotrophoblast lacunae providing a rich source of nutrition for the embryo. The intervillous space is derived from these networks and is fed by maternal blood which enters via 80–100 spiral arteries.
- The terminal villi of the placenta are constantly bathed in maternal blood within the interillous spaces, and this arrangement provides for an extremely large area for the exchange of metabolic and gaseous products between the maternal and fetal bloodstreams. There is normally no intermingling of blood between these two compartments.
- Normal physiological placental vascular adaptation in pregnancy involves conversion of the muscular walls of the maternal spiral arteries into large low pressure capacitance vessels, which can accommodate the massive increase in blood flow that the feto-placental unit requires.
- Cytotrophoblast invasion into the spiral arteries (endovascular invasion) leads to the loss of the endothelial lining and most, if not all, of the musculoelastic tissue. By the end of the second trimester, the maternal spiral arteries are lined exclusively by cytotrophoblasts, and endothelial cells are no longer present in either the endometrial or myometrial segments.

Vasa previa

- Vasa previa occurs when fetal vessels run through the membranes below the fetal presenting part and close to the internal cervical os. There is usually no protection in the form of Wharton's jelly.
- Risk factors include multiple pregnancy, velamentous cord insertion, and the presence of succenturiate or accessory lobes.
- The danger is fetal exsanguination when the membranes rupture spontaneously or when ruptured artificially. Unless the diagnosis is suspected, fetal death can occur very rapidly. The diagnosis should be entertained in the presense of heavy vaginal bleeding and fetal heart rate abnormalities. The sinusoidal heart rate pattern is a relatively late phenomenon.
- The diagnosis is easily made on prenatal ultrasound using colour Doppler. If vessels are seen crossing the internal os, the diagnosis should be obvious. Planned Caesarean section is the recommended mode of delivery.

Chorioangioma

- Chorioangiomas are benign vascular tumors of the placenta. They are the most common primary tumors of the placenta. On ultrasound, a hyperechoic mass near the placental cord insertion site is seen.
- Chorioangiomas can function as an arteriovenous shunt causing fetal anemia, non-immune hydrops, and polyhydramnios. Most cases are detected only after routine placental pathology. In general, pregnancy complications are rare with lesions <6 cm in diameter. There is usually no associated fetal structural malformations.
- There is no specific fetal intervention. Monitoring is, however, required to detect the development of cardiac failure, polyhydramnios, and hydrops. Preterm labor secondary to polyhydramnios may complicate the pregnancy.

Umbilical cord abnormalities

- These include abnormal number of vessels, short cord, cord cysts, hyper- or hypocoiled cord, hemangiomas, aneurysms, etc.
- The diagnosis is usually made on ultrasound. The fetal prognosis very much depends on the presence of other structural malformations. Various chromosome abnormalities have been reported in association with umbilical cord malformations.
- The umbilical cord grows as a result of fetal movement throughout pregnancy. Short umbilical cords have been associated with the fetal akinesia syndrome and limb–body wall complex abnormalities.
- Adverse perinatal outcome is associated with abnormalities of umbilical cord coiling. Cords which are hypocoiled are associated with fetal heart rate abnormalities in labor. Preterm labor and delivery, fetal growth restriction, and low birth weight have been reported with hypercoiled cords.
- Although the degree of umbilical cord coiling is generally not part of the routine mid trimester fetal anomaly scan, if an abnormality is detected, consideration should be given for serial monitoring if possible.

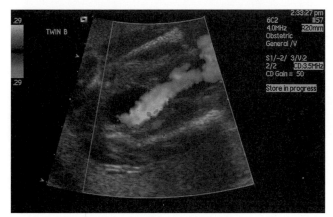

Fig. 19.1. Single umbilical artery. See color plate section.

Single umbilical artery (SUA)

- The umbilical cord contains two arteries and one vein. SUA (Fig. 19.1) is found in approximately 1% of normal newborns, but the incidence doubles if congenital malformations are present.
- SUA can arise secondary to primary agenesis of either the right or left vessel, atresia of a previously normal vessel or persistence of the original allantoic artery of the body stalk.
- The left artery is reported to be absent more frequently than the right.
- Malformations including the ADAMS complex, multicystic renal dysplasia, Potter sequence, sirenomelia, cardiac defects, renal anomalies, genitourinary defects, limb deficiencies, intestinal atresias, imperforate anus, VACTERL syndrome, etc. are all more frequently observed in babies with SUA.
- There is also an association with fetal growth restriction and preterm delivery.
- If the abnormality is detected antenatally, careful evaluation of the fetus for additional structural malformations should be performed. Karyotyping is indicated if additional anomalies are detected. Serial growth scans may be considered in view of the association with intrauterine growth restriction.

19

PLACENTA, UMBILICAL CORD ABNORMALITIES

20

FETAL HYDROPS

Hydrops

- Hydrops is an end-stage process for a number of fetal diseases resulting in tissue edema and/or fluid collection (ascites, pleural effusion, pericardial effusion) in various sites (Fig. 20.1).
- Its etiology may be either immune or non-immune depending on the presence or absence of red cell alloimmunization. Non-immune causes now account for 90% of all cases of hydrops.
- The most common causes associated with hydrops are congenital heart abnormalities, abnormalities in heart rate, twin-to-twin transfusion syndrome, congenital anomalies, aneuploidy, infections, congenital anemia, and congenital chylothorax (Table 20.1).
- Extravascular accumulation of fluid may occur as a result of decreased intravascular osmotic pressure, increased intravascular hydrostatic pressure, or aberrations in lymphatic flow.
- Hypoalbuminemia may cause low intravascular oncotic pressure. Hypoxic mediated endothelial damage may result in leaking of albumin into the interstitial space. Fetal liver dysfunction (in chronically anemic fetuses with increased extramedullary erythropoiesis or portal hypertension) can also result in decreased hepatic production of proteins that result in reduced intravascular oncotic pressure.
- Fetal cardiac dysfunction or increased intrathoracic pressure (because of lung masses or effusions) can lead to increased central venous pressure and delayed lymphatic drainage, which results in the development of hydrops. In most cases the cause of hydrops is multifactorial.
- Regardless of the etiology, hydrops has a very poor outcome (>80% mortality) despite improvements in diagnosis and management. Early development of hydrops has a particularly poor prognosis.
- The mortality rate is highest among neonates with congenital anomalies (60%) and lowest among neonates with congenital chylothorax (6%). Mortality is higher in premature infants and those delivered in poor condition (lower 5-minute Apgar scores, higher levels of inspired oxygen support, and more often treated with high-frequency ventilation during the first day after birth).
- Once the diagnosis is made, urgent referral to a fetal medicine unit is essential.
- It is important to obtain a detailed family, medical, obstetric, and genetic history. Consider prior exposure to possible viral infections (maternal rash, arthralgia/myalgia) should also be specifically excluded.
- Detailed ultrasound performed to detect structural abnormalities, particularly cardiac and thoracic abnormalities. The umbilical cord and placenta should be carefully examined to exclude vascular malformations. Fetal heart rate and rhythm should be examined to exclude fetal tachy- or brady-arrhythmias.

20

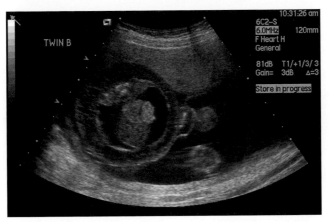

Fig. 20.1. Hydrops with skin edema and ascites.

- Maternal blood should be taken for full viral screen (CMV, parvovirus, rubella, herpes), toxoplasma serology, blood group and antibody screen, and hemoglobin electrophoresis.
- Fetal anemia should be excluded by middle cerebral artery peak systolic velocity monitoring. Fetal echocardiography should be performed in all cases.
- If anemia is suspected, the most likely cause is parvovirus infection. This is a treatable condition with usually a one off fetal transfusion. There are minimal long-term sequelae.
- Karyotyping is mandatory in all cases. Amniocentesis is the method of choice unless anemia is suspected. Samples should be sent for cytogenetics and infection screen using PCR.
- If hydrops is secondary to fetal arrhythmia, consider maternal therapy. Occasionally, direct fetal treatment may be required in cases of fetal supraventricular tachycardia unresponsive to maternal treatment.
- If the hydrops is secondary to a structural anomaly (e.g. pleural effusion), in utero therapy (pleuroamniotic shunting) may be necessary.
- Offer termination of pregnancy if hydrops is severe, presence of major malformations, or aneuploidy. Counsel parents that untreated hydrops carries a very high (>80%) perinatal mortality rate and that outcome is likely to be poor.
- Postmortem essential to help with diagnosis and predict risk of recurrence. Not infrequently, evidence of viral infection detected on histopathology, despite negative maternal and fetal testing.
- Refer for genetic counseling if appropriate.

20

Table 20.1

Cardiovascular
Hypoplastic left heart
Hypoplastic right heart
A-V canal defects
Premature closure of foramen ovale
Transposition of the great vessels
Ebstein's anomaly
Atrial flutter
Supraventricular tachycardia
Complete heart block
Placental chorioangioma
Sacrococcygeal teratoma
Umbilical cord hemangioma
Twin pregnancy
Twin–twin transfusion syndrome
Acardiac twin
Chromosomal
Trisomy 13, 18, 21
Triploidy
Thoracic
Congenital cystic adenomatoid malformation
Diaphragmatic hernia
Pulmonary sequestration
Primary hydrothorax
Bronchogenic cyst
Intrathoracic mass
Haematologic
Alpha-thalassemia
Feto-maternal hemorrhage
Red cell enzyme deficiencies

Table 20.1 (*cont.*)

Infections
Parvovirus B19
Cytomegalovirus
Syphilis
Herpes
Rubella
Genetic syndromes
Arthrogryposis
Lethal multiple pterygium syndrome
Pena–Shokeir syndrome
Myotonic dystrophy
Metabolic disorders
Gangliosidosis
Galactosialidosis
Gaucher's disease

- Neonatology input is needed, particularly if delivery is considered an option. Cesarean section probably better as most hydropic fetuses are unable to tolerate the stress of vaginal delivery. Long-term outcome may not be altered with abdominal delivery. The combination of severe hydrops and prematurity carries a particularly poor prognosis.

INDEX

INDEX